AUTOIMMUNE FIX
DIET
COOKBOOK:

Recipes that will help Prevent Hidden Autoimmune Damages and Keep you Living Healthy.

By

Brain Thompson

Disclaimer:

The information provided in this book is designed to provide helpful information on the subjects discussed. The publisher and author are not responsible for any specific health or allergy needs that may require medical supervision and are not liable for any damages or negative consequences from any treatment, action, application or preparation, to any person reading or following the information in this book.

Table of Contents

Introduction:

Rise up and stop the hidden autoimmune damages that keeps you sick, fat, and tired before it get it escalates

The blood cells in the body's immune system help in protecting your body against harmful substances. Examples include viruses, cancer cells, bacteria, toxins, and blood and tissue from outside the body. These substances contain antigens and immune system produces antibodies against these antigens that enable it to destroy these harmful substances.

However, when you have an autoimmune disorder, your immune system does not differentiate between healthy tissue and antigens. By so doing, the body sets off a reaction that destroys normal tissues.

Furthermore, the exact cause of autoimmune disorders is unknown to man. One theory is that some microorganisms (like bacteria or viruses) or drugs may cause changes that confuse the immune system. This often happen in people who have genes that make them more prone to autoimmune disorders.

According to the American Autoimmune Related Diseases Association (AARDA) millions of people suffer from autoimmunity whether they know it or not. The major cause of most weight gain, brain and mood problems, and fatigue, autoimmunity can take years—for symptoms and a clear diagnosis to arise.

In addition, through years of research, Dr. Tom O'Bryan has discovered that autoimmunity is actually a spectrum, and large numbers of people experiencing general malaise are already on it. Autoimmune diseases, such as Alzheimer's, osteoporosis, Multiple Sclerosis, diabetes, and lupus, have become the third leading cause of death behind heart disease and cancer, a large number of people affected are left in the dark.

Finally, the good news is that many autoimmune conditions can be reversed permanently through a targeted protocol designed to heal the autoimmune system, 70 percent of which is located in the gut.

The Autoimmune Fix Diet Cookbook includes recipes that will keep you living healthy with chronic illness. The meals are categorized into beverages, beef and pork, dessert, appetizer and much more. In the first 3 weeks, I suggest you follow a Paleo-inspired diet during which you cut out gluten, sweets, and dairy (the three primary culprits behind autoimmunity). This cookbook will help you fix the dietary aspect and focus on the other causes of autoimmunity such as genetics and microbiome. *The Autoimmune Fix* Diet Cookbook provides a practical and much-needed guide to navigating these increasingly common conditions to help you feel better and develop a plan that works for you.

Recipes that will help Prevent Hidden Autoimmune Damages and Keep you Living Healthy.

Appetizer & Snacks

Cucumber and Dill Summer Soup
Serves: 4-8

Ingredients

1 avocado (pitted and peeled)

½ cup of filtered water

1 tablespoon fresh, chopped basil

Juice from one lemon

2 cucumbers (peeled and chopped)

1 cup of full-fat coconut milk

3 tablespoons of fresh, chopped dill

1 teaspoon of grated lemon zest

½ teaspoon of sea salt

Note: I suggest you reserve some cucumber, avocado, dill, and lemon.

Directions:

1. First, you puree all ingredients in blender or food processor until smooth.
2. Then for extra smooth soup, I advise you pour through fine mesh sieve to filter out extra vegetable fibers.
3. Finally, you chill and serve with shredded chicken or shrimp as main dish or garnished as appetizer.

Raw Citrus Poke Salad

Serves: 4

Ingredients

½ small head cauliflower (chopped into florets)

½ large cucumbers (chopped)

1 tablespoon of lemon juice

1 tablespoon of white wine vinegar

1 tablespoon of fish sauce

½ teaspoon of powdered ginger

Cilantro sprigs (to garnish)

1 lb. of sushi-grade salmon or better still ahi tuna, boneless and skinless (I used salmon, but either is fine)

1 avocado (cubed)

4 green onions, sliced thin (I suggest you reserve small amount for garnish)

1 tablespoon of lime juice

1 tablespoon of coconut aminos

1 tablespoon of olive oil

¼ teaspoon of garlic powder

Directions:

1. First, you use a very sharp knife, cut fish into roughly 1-inch cubes and place in large bowl.
2. After which you add avocado, cucumber, and green onion to fish.
3. After that, you place cauliflower into food processor and pulse just until processed into "rice" sized grains; set-aside.
4. At this point, you whisk last eight ingredients in a separate bowl to combine.
5. This is when you pour into bowl of fish and vegetables.
6. Then you mix gently to coat fish and vegetables in sauce.
7. Finally, you refrigerate to chill and marinate for about 20 minutes.

8. Make sure you serve over raw cauliflower "rice."

NOTE: remember that it is very important to follow guidelines on using raw fish, to purchase sushi-grade quality, and to work closely with your fishmonger to ensure safety.

BBQ Chicken Meatballs

Serves: 4 servings

Ingredients

¼ cup AIP-friendly barbecue sauce

2 tablespoons of cooking fat

1 lb. of ground chicken

¼ cup of cilantro (chopped)

¼ cup of red onion (chopped)

Directions:

1. First, you combine the chicken, barbecue sauce, cilantro, and red onion and form into 1-inch balls.
2. After which you heat the cooking fat in a skillet over medium heat.
3. Then you sauté the meatballs until cooked through, about 10-15 minutes, stirring occasionally.

Roasted Garlic Cauliflower Hummus

Serves: 3 cups

Ingredients

½ teaspoon of coconut oil

½ cup of extra virgin olive oil

2 tablespoons of water

1 head of garlic

1 head of cauliflower (steamed)

1 lemon (juiced)

½ teaspoon of sea salt

Parsley, green olives, and additional olive oil to serve

Directions:

1. Meanwhile, you heat your oven to 400 degrees.
2. After which you cut the very top off of the head of garlic, making sure to expose the tip of every clove.
3. After that, you place the coconut oil on the top and wrap in foil.
4. At this point, you cook in the oven for 30 minutes, or until soft and lightly browned.
5. Then when the garlic is finished roasting, remove the cloves and place in a food processor with the cauliflower, olive oil, lemon juice, water, and sea salt.
6. This is when you process for a minute or two, until a thick puree forms.
7. Finally, you serve garnished with parsley, green olives, and olive oil.

Meatballs in Sticky Peach Sauce

Serves: 4 to 6 servings

Ingredients

1 pound of ground pork

1 tablespoon of minced fresh rosemary

¾ teaspoon of fine sea salt

1 pound of ground beef

3 tablespoons of no-sugar-added peach preserves (preferably homemade or store-bought)

1 teaspoon of dried thyme leaves

Directions:

1. First, you combine all meatball ingredients together in a large mixing bowl with your hands until evenly distributed.
2. After which you form 2-tablepoon-sized meatballs and place directly in a large skillet set over the stovetop.
3. Remember that you will be able to fit the most meatballs if you place them in a concentric pattern.
4. Then once all the meatballs have been placed in the skillet, turn the heat to medium-high.
5. At this point, you cook for about 6 minutes until browned on the bottom, turn over with a spoon and cook an additional 5 to 6 minutes until slightly pink in the center.
6. This is when you turn off the heat and stir the meatballs to coat them in the pan juices.
7. Furthermore, you spoon the Sticky Peach Sauce on top of the meatballs.
8. After that, you broil for about 4 to 5 minutes until the sauce has caramelized.
9. Finally, you serve warm over mashed parsnips or white sweet potatoes with the sauce spooned on top!

Sticky Peach Sauce

Serves: ½ cup

Ingredients

⅓ Cup of chicken broth

½ teaspoon of orange zest

Pinch of sea salt

1 tablespoon of cold water

½ cup of no-sugar-added peach preserves (preferably homemade or store-bought)

3 tablespoons of fresh-squeezed orange juice

3 large of Medjool dates (pitted)

2 teaspoons of arrowroot starch

Directions:

1. First, you combine the preserves, broth, juice, and zest in a small saucepan over medium-high heat.
2. Then while you wait for the mixture to come to a boil, cover dates in a small dish with water and microwave for about 30 to 60 seconds until softened.
3. After that, you drain the water and mash the dates into a paste using a fork.
4. At this point, once the mixture has been boiling and reducing down for 5 to 7 minutes until thickened, whisk in the date paste and sea salt until well combined.
5. This is when you remove from heat.
6. Furthermore, you whisk together the arrowroot and cold water in a small dish and then pour directly into the saucepan.
7. Finally, you whisk continuously for 1 minute to thicken the sauce (NOTE: it will lighten up in color and thicken to a sticky sauce).

Holiday Stuffed Mushroom Appetizer

Serves: 24

Ingredients

1 tablespoon of solid cooking fat (melted)

¼ cup of minced shallot

¼ cup of packed fresh parsley

2 teaspoons of white wine

24 cremini mushrooms (cleaned)

½ lb. of ground pork

4 garlic cloves (minced)

1 teaspoon of sea salt

Directions:

1. Meanwhile, you heat oven to 450 degrees F.
2. After which you line a baking sheet with foil or parchment paper.
3. After that, you snap the stem off each mushroom, leaving a well in the cap.
4. At this point, you set the stems aside.
5. This is when you toss the mushrooms in the melted fat.
6. Furthermore, you place them cap up on the baking sheet.
7. After which you roast them for 10 minutes in the hot oven.
8. After that, you flip each mushroom and roast for another 10 minutes.
9. Then while mushrooms are roasting, you place shallot, garlic, parsley, and mushroom stems in food processor.
10. In addition, you pulse to combine mixture.
11. Combine the pork and salt with the veggie mixture in a large bowl.
12. After that, you stuff each mushroom well with a generous spoon of pork filling.
13. Then you place stuffed mushrooms back on sheet and sprinkle with wine.
14. Finally, you roast for another 12 minutes or until filling is slightly browned on top.
15. Then you serve hot.

Notes

1. Remember that it is okay to cook with alcohol during the elimination phase of AIP.
2. You should have in mind that the alcohol will cook off. If you'd rather skip the wine though, the recipe will still turn out great.

Pumpkin Spice Granola

Serves: 6 servings

Ingredients

⅔ Cup of raisins

2 medium bananas with brown spots

1 ½ teaspoon of cinnamon

¼ teaspoon of sea salt

2 cups of unsweetened coconut flakes

⅔ Cup of chopped apple rings

2 tablespoons of melted coconut oil

1 teaspoon of ground ginger

½ teaspoon of ground mace

Directions:

1. Meanwhile, you heat oven to 300 degrees F.
2. After which you line a baking sheet with parchment paper or grease well with coconut oil.
3. After that, you stir together coconut flakes, raisins, and apple rings in a medium mixing bowl.
4. Then in a separate medium bowl, you mash the banana until smooth ensuring you have ⅔ cup of mash.
5. At this point, you stir the coconut oil, spices, and sea salt into the mashed banana.
6. This is when you coat the dry mixture with the wet mixture by stirring until well combined and everything sticks together.
7. Furthermore, you spread out evenly onto prepared baking sheet into a ¼-inch layer.
8. After that, you bake for about 45 to 50 minutes, stirring halfway through, until the granola is a golden brown and smells of baked pumpkin bread.
9. Finally, you let cool for at least 10 to 15 minutes to set.
10. Make sure you break any large chunks into smaller, bite-sized pieces.

Shopping tip:

Remember, these may be labeled coconut chips in the bulk bins at health food stores.

Kale Pesto
Serves: 2 cups

Ingredients

¾ cup of extra virgin olive oil

½ teaspoon of sea salt

1 bunch kale, chopped (preferably about 4 cups, packed)

1 lemon (juiced)

2-3 cloves of garlic

Directions:

1. First, you add all of the ingredients to a high-powered blender or a food processor.
2. After which you blend or process for about 30 seconds or until a paste forms.
3. Then you use a tamper, or stop periodically to scrape down the sides of the processor once or twice.

Notes

Storage: you can keep in the refrigerator for about a week.

Lox & Everything Sweet Potatoes

Serves: 10-12

Ingredients

1 recipe Onion and Dill "Cream Cheese"

Fresh dill (for serving)

1 recipe Everything Sweet Potatoes

4 oz. of AIP-compliant smoked salmon

Directions:

1. First, you top cooled sweet potatoes with a layer of smoked salmon, a dollop of "Cream Cheese" and a few pieces of fresh dill.
2. Then you serve immediately or place in the refrigerator for up to a day to serve cold.

Bacon-Wrapped Cinnamon Apples

Serves: 20

Ingredients

1 teaspoon of cinnamon

1 teaspoon of chopped thyme (or better still ½ teaspoon of dried thyme)

2 organic apples

6-8 slices of bacon

Directions:

1. Meanwhile, you heat the oven to 350 degrees.
2. After which you line a baking sheet with parchment paper.
3. After that, you prepare your apples by coring and slicing them into ½-inch pieces.
4. Then you coat evenly with cinnamon in a mixing bowl.
5. At this point, you slice the bacon crosswise into thirds so that the pieces are long enough to be wrapped around the apples once.
6. This is when you proceed with wrapping one slice of bacon around one apple slice, and placing seam side down on the baking sheet.
7. Furthermore, you bake on the middle oven rack for about 23-25 minutes until the apples are softened.
8. After that, you broil for about 3 minutes until the bacon begins to caramelize.
9. Finally, you let cool before serving.
10. Make sure you secure with toothpicks if serving as a party appetizer.

Shrimp Ceviche Salad

Serves: 2 servings

Ingredients

1 ½ cups of chopped green apple

1 cup of chopped cooked shrimp

2 tablespoons of finely chopped mint

2 tablespoons of lemon juice

¼ teaspoon of garlic powder

1 ½ cups of seeded and chopped cucumber

Meat of 1 avocado (diced)

¼ cup of parsley (finely chopped)

2 tablespoons of olive oil

½ teaspoon of sea salt

Directions:

1. First, you mix all ingredients together in a serving bowl.
2. Then you refrigerate for at least two hours to let flavors marry.
3. Finally, you stir well before serving.

Cherry-Ginger Gummies

Serves: 24 gummies

Ingredients

¾ cup of water

¼ cup of maple syrup

¼ cup of gelatin

3 tablespoon of lemon juice

1 cup of fresh (or better still frozen cherries)

1 teaspoon of powdered ginger

Directions:

1. First, you pour lemon juice, water, and cherries into blender and blend on high until smooth.
2. After which you pour mixture into saucepan.
3. After that, you turn heat to medium-low and whisk in maple syrup, ginger, and gelatin.
4. At this point, you continue to whisk for about 5 minutes, until the mixture is thin and there are no clumps.
5. If you using a mold, I suggest you place mold on baking sheet for ease of transfer to refrigerator.

Note: carefully pour mixture into mold or baking dish.

6. Then you set in refrigerator to firm for 1 hour.
7. On the other hand if you using a mold, I suggest you transfer to freezer for 5 minutes (set a timer!) in order to easily pop gummies from the mold (NOTE: If using a baking dish, cut into squares).

Hard Cider and Maple Brined Pork Belly

Serves: 4-6

Ingredients

¼ cup of sea salt

One cinnamon stick

1½ - 2 lbs. of pork belly

24 oz. of hard apple cider

3 tablespoons of maple syrup

One 1-inch piece fresh ginger (peeled and chopped)

1 bay leaf

Directions:

1. First, you place pork in the freezer while making brine (**NOTE:** about 5 minutes, makes scoring fat easier).
2. After which you combine all ingredients, except pork belly, in a pot over medium heat.
3. After that, you bring to simmer, stirring until salt dissolves.
4. Then when brine begins to simmer, remove from heat.
5. At this point, you allow cooling completely in refrigerator.
6. This is when you remove pork from freezer, using sharp knife; score fat in diamond pattern.
7. Furthermore, you place pork in gallon-size sealable bag, pour cooled brine in bag, seal, place in large bowl.
8. After which you allow to brine in refrigerator overnight or for 8 hours.
9. Meanwhile, you heat oven to 250 degrees F.
10. After that, you remove pork from brine, discard liquid.
11. In addition, you place pork, fat cap up, on rack in roasting pan.
12. At this point, you roast for about 1 hour, 30 minutes.
13. At the 1-hour mark, I suggest you start checking pork every 10 minutes to make sure it is not overcooked.
14. Then when finished roasting, turn broiler to low.
15. This is when you broil pork for about 3-4 minutes (watch carefully) or until fat is browned and very crispy.
16. Finally, you remove from oven, slice with serrated knife as soon as it is cool enough to handle.

17. Then you serve warm.

Notes

Remember that I have not tried this substitute for the hard cider, but if you'd like to use non-alcohol brine, I would experiment with roughly 2 cups water, ¾ cup apple juice, and ¼ cup apple cider vinegar.

Prosciutto Meatloaf Muffins with Fig Jam
Serves: 12 muffins

Ingredients

2 lbs. of ground beef

5 oz. of AIP-friendly prosciutto

½ teaspoon of sea salt

2 cups of white sweet potato (cubed)

1 tablespoon of thyme leaves

½ teaspoon of granulated garlic

Directions:

1. Meanwhile, you heat oven to 350 degrees F.
2. After which you line 12 muffin cups with prosciutto slices ensuring the sides and bottom are covered.
3. After that, you set a steamer basket over a pot of boiling water.
4. Then you place sweet potatoes in the basket, cover, and let steam cook for about 10-12 minutes until the potatoes easily break apart with a fork.
5. At this point, you place cooked sweet potatoes, beef, thyme leaves, and sea salt in a high-powered blender or food processor.
6. This is when you process until the sweet potatoes and meat are pureed into a paste.
7. Furthermore, you spoon ⅓ cup of the meatloaf mixture into each prosciutto-lined muffin cup.
8. After that, you bake on the middle rack of the oven for 23 minutes.
9. Then you spoon 1 tablespoon of Fig Jam on top of each muffin and broil on high for 2-3 minutes until the jam begins to caramelize.
10. Finally, you remove and serve warm with extra Fig Jam on the side.

Fig Jam

Serves: 1 cup

Ingredients

¼ cup of orange Juice

1 teaspoon of orange zest

Pinch of sea salt

1 cup of dried black mission figs (stems removed)

2 sprigs of thyme

¼ teaspoon of cinnamon

1 tablespoon of apple cider vinegar

Directions:

1. First, you place the dried figs, orange juice, thyme sprigs, and enough water to barely cover the figs in your smallest saucepan.
2. After which you bring to a boil, cover, and lower the heat to maintain a simmer for 20 minutes.
3. After that, you place figs, remaining water from the pot, and the rest of the Fig Jam ingredients in a blender or food processor.
4. Finally, you blend on low speed until a jam-like consistency has formed, about 30 seconds.

Lemon-Raspberry Gelatin Gummies
Serves: 24 gummies

Ingredients

1 cup of frozen raspberries

¼ cup of grass-fed gelatin (I prefer this brand)

Directions:

1. First, you place lemon juice and raspberries in a blender and blend on high until completely mixed.
2. After which you pour into a saucepan.
3. After that, you add the honey and gelatin and whisk together (NOTE: You will have a thick paste).
4. Then you turn the heat on low, and continue to whisk the mixture for about 5-10 minutes, until it becomes thin and everything is incorporated.
5. At this point, you take off the heat.
6. This is when you pour into silicone molds or a small baking dish.
7. Furthermore, you set in the refrigerator for at least 1 hour to firm up.
8. If you used a small baking dish as a receptacle, I suggest you cut into bite-size squares. Otherwise, remove gummies from their molds and enjoy!

Garlic Rosemary Plantain Crackers

Serves: 2 cups

Ingredients

½ cup of coconut oil (melted)

½ teaspoon of sea salt

2 large, green plantains

2 tablespoons of fresh rosemary (chopped)

1 teaspoon of granulated garlic

Directions:

1. Meanwhile, you heat the oven to 300 degrees F.
2. After which you cut a slit from one end to the other of the plantains and use that cut to peel them.
3. After that you chop them into large chunks and place them in a high-powered blender or food processor with the coconut oil, rosemary, garlic, and sea salt.
4. Then you blend or process until a slightly thick and chunky mixture forms.
5. At this point, you pour out onto a baking sheet lined with parchment paper and smooth out until it is a ¼" thick with either a spatula or another piece of parchment paper and a rolling pin.
6. This is when you bake in the oven for 10 minutes.
7. Furthermore, you remove and score into 1½" crackers with a knife.
8. Finally, you place back into the oven and cook for another 50 minutes to 1-hour.

NOTE that they are finished cooking when the crackers are a nice medium brown and the ones in the middle are no longer soft.

Remember that you may need to cook these up to 20 minutes more to let them get fully crispy.

Have at the back of your mind that crackers keep sealed in an airtight container for a week or so (if you don't eat them sooner than that!)

Serves: 4

Ingredients

1 cup of water

4-5 pounds of baby artichokes

4 slices of sugar-free (pastured bacon)

1 lemon (juiced)

Directions:

1. First, you cook the bacon slices in a cast-iron skillet on medium-low heat, turning a few times and cooking until they are nice and crispy (about 10-15 minutes depending on thickness).
2. Then while the bacon is cooking, prep the artichokes.
3. After that, you place the water and lemon juice in a medium sized bowl and set aside.
4. If you want to prep the artichokes, I suggest you take off a majority of the outer leaves, until all of the leaves are soft and edible besides the very top.
5. After which you slice off the top portion, and cut in half.
6. At this point, you place prepped halves in the bowl with lemon water, which prevents them from turning brown before you go to cook them.
7. This is when you repeat this process with all of the artichokes.
8. When the bacon is finished cooking, you set it aside, leaving the fat in the pan.
9. Furthermore, you turn the heat up to medium-high and add the artichokes.
10. In addition, you sauté for 10 minutes, stirring, until cooked throughout and browned on the edges.
11. Finally, you crumble or chop the bacon into bits and serve warm with them on top.

Bacon-Beef Liver Pâté with Rosemary and Thyme

Serves: 2 cups

Ingredients

1 small onion (minced)

1 pound of grass-fed beef liver

2 tablespoons of fresh thyme (minced)

Slices of fresh carrot or better still cucumber

6 pieces of uncured bacon

4 cloves garlic (minced)

2 tablespoons of fresh rosemary (minced)

½ cup of coconut oil (melted)

½ teaspoon of sea salt

Directions:

1. First, you cook the bacon slices in a cast-iron pot until crispy.
2. After which you set aside to cool, reserving the grease in the pan to cook the liver.
3. After that, you add the onion and cook for about 2 minutes on medium-high.
4. At this point, you add the garlic and cook for a minute.
5. This is when you add the liver, sprinkling with the herbs.
6. Then you cook for about 3-5 minutes per side, until no longer pink in the center.
7. Furthermore, you turn off heat, and place contents into a blender or food processor or with the coconut oil and sea salt.
8. After which you process until it forms a thick paste, adding more coconut oil if too thick.
9. Finally, you cut the cooled bacon strips into little bits and mix with the pâté in a small bowl.
10. Make sure you garnish with some fresh herbs and serve on carrot or cucumber slices.

Roasted Beet Dip
Serves: 6

Ingredients

1 tablespoon of coconut oil (melted)

¼ cup of water

1 lemon (juiced)

½ teaspoon of salt

2 pounds beets (peeled and cut into chunks)

⅓ Cup of extra-virgin olive oil

1 tablespoon of apple- cider vinegar

2 cloves garlic (peeled)

Directions:

1. Meanwhile, you heat your oven to 400 degrees.
2. After which you arrange the beets in a baking dish and coat with the coconut oil.
3. After that, you bake for 1 hour or until tender, stirring every 20 minutes.
4. This is when you let the beets cool for 10 minutes and then place them in a blender or food processor with the olive oil, water, apple-cider vinegar, lemon juice, garlic, and salt.
5. Then you blend until a thick paste forms, if it is too thick add more olive oil one tablespoon at a time.
6. Finally, you serve on fresh vegetable slices.

Sweet Potato Fries with Garlic "Mayo"

Tips:

Remember that the "Mayo" must cool at room temperature for an hour or in the refrigerator for 20 minutes.

Serves: 4-6

Ingredients

<u>Ingredients for the "Mayo":</u>

1/2 cup of warm filtered water

1/4 teaspoon of salt

1/2 cup coconut concentrate, slightly warmed

1/4 cup of extra-virgin olive oil

3-4 cloves garlic

<u>Ingredients for the Fries:</u>

4 tablespoons of solid cooking fat (melted)

3 large sweet potatoes (peeled and cut into thick fries)

Sea salt to taste

Directions:

<u>Directions on how to make the mayo:</u>

1. First, you place the coconut concentrate, warm water, olive oil, garlic cloves and salt in a blender and blend on high for a minute or two, until the sauce thickens.
2. After which you let cool for an hour at room temperature – alternately, you can place it in the refrigerator for about 20 minutes.
3. If you would like to use the sauce in a cold dish, I suggest you thin with water until the desired consistency are reached.

<u>Directions on how to make the fries:</u>

1. Meanwhile, you heat your oven to 400 degrees.
2. After which you place the sweet potato fries into a large bowl and coat with the cooking fat and sea salt.

3. After that, you arrange on a series of baking sheets so that the fries have adequate space between them (this is how they come out crispy).
4. Then you use 3-4 sheets if you need to! Add the sea salt.
5. Finally, you bake for about 10-15 minutes, remove from the oven, flip, and bake for another 10-15 minutes, watching at the end so that they don't burn.

Note: Remember, "Mayo" well in the refrigerator, but hardens. Let come to room-temperature or warm gently before using.

Green Detox Smoothie

Serves: 2 large or 4 small glasses

Ingredients

1 kiwi (peeled and roughly sliced)

¼ packed cup curly parsley (stalks included)

2 cups of coconut water

1 Granny Smith apple (cored and roughly chopped, peel left on)

1 large green kale leaf, stalk removed (you can save it for something else), leaf roughly chopped

2½-inch piece cucumber (thickly sliced, peel left on)

¾-inch piece fresh ginger (peeled and sliced)

Directions:

1. First, you put all the ingredients into a high speed blender and blend until completely smooth.

Egg-less Nog!

Serves: 4

Ingredients

2½ cups of coconut milk

¼ teaspoon of cinnamon powder

Pinch of sea salt

Pinch mace

½ cup of pumpkin purée

½ teaspoon of alcohol-free vanilla extract

1 tablespoon of maple syrup

¼ teaspoon of gelatin

Directions:

1. First, you put the pumpkin purée, coconut milk, vanilla extract, cinnamon powder, maple syrup and sea salt into a medium pan and heat to just below simmering.
2. After which you remove from the heat and sprinkle in the gelatin, whisking thoroughly until melted and the liquid is frothy.
3. After that, you allow to cool slightly (**NOTE:** the gelatin will not set the drink; it is there to thicken it slightly).
4. Then you pour into 4 glasses, let cool and then refrigerate until needed.
5. This is when you add a sprinkling of mace before serving.

Pomegranate Cider

Serves: 2 servings

Ingredients

1 cup of apple juice

2 inches fresh ginger (peeled and sliced)

2 cups of pomegranate juice

1 cinnamon stick

1 whole clove

Directions:

1. First, in a small saucepan over medium heat, combine all ingredients and bring to a simmer.
2. Then you simmer for 10 minutes, then strain and serve.

Watermelon-Basil Shrub (A Drink!)
Serves: Approx. 16

Ingredients

1 large bunch basil (chopped)

½ cup of white balsamic vinegar

Ice

½ medium watermelon, cubed, rind removed (at approx. 5-6 cups)

½ cup of honey

Sparkling mineral water

Directions:

1. First, you crush and mix melon, basil, and honey in large, glass bowl or jar.
2. After which you cover tightly and allow macerating in refrigerator for about 2-3 days.
3. After that, you pour fruit mixture into blender and process until smooth.
4. Then you strain through cheesecloth to remove seeds and pulp. (**NOTE:** You should have approx. 2½-3 cups juice.)
5. At this point, you mix juice with vinegar.
6. This is when you pour ¼-1/2 cup each in bottom of serving glasses, depending on the flavor strength you like.
7. Finally, you fill glass with ice and add sparkling water to fill.
8. Serve and enjoy!

Notes

Remember that the syrup will keep in refrigerator, ready to add to drinks, for several weeks.

Berry-Infused Thai Drinking Vinegar

Serves: 16 servings

Ingredients

1 cup of blackberries

Sparkling water (for serving)

2 cups of apple cider vinegar

1 cup of raspberries

½ - 1 cup of honey

Directions:

1. First, you combine the vinegar and berries in a 1-quart jar with an airtight lid (NOTE: as for me, I used a 1-quart mason jar with a plastic screw-on cap).
2. After which you let sit for seven days at room temperature.
3. After that, you strain out the fruit and pour the vinegar back into the jar.
4. Then you add honey and shake well.
5. Furthermore, you refrigerate for seven more days, shaking occasionally to help dissolve the honey.
6. If you want to serve, I suggest you place one ounce of the drinking vinegar in a 16-ounce glass.
7. Make sure you fill the glass with ice and then top off with sparkling water.
8. Then you stir to combine.

Creamy Coconut Milk

Serves: 12 ounces

Ingredients

2 cups of boiling water

Sea salt (to taste)

1 cup of unsweetened coconut flakes (I prefer this variety)

Blender

Cheesecloth

Directions:

1. First, you place the shredded coconut and boiling water in your blender and blend on high speed for a few minutes, taking breaks for the motor if needed.
2. After which you let cool for at least 15 minutes-until it can be safely handled.
3. Then you strain through cheesecloth into a glass jar.

Collagen-Berry Green Smoothie

Serves: 1

Ingredients

¼ cup of water

1 tablespoon coconut concentrate

Ice cubes (optional to taste)

1 banana

½ cup of frozen berries

1 tablespoon of collagen

1 cup of spinach

Directions:

1. First, you place all ingredients in a blender and blend to combine.
2. After which you add ice cubes if smoothie is not cold or thick enough.
3. Then you enjoy immediately.

Anti-Inflammatory Turmeric Tea

Serves: 4

Ingredients

½ Tablespoon of turmeric powder

1 handful cilantro (chopped)

1 Tablespoon of olive oil

1 orange, juiced (or better still substitute 1½ tablespoon honey)

32 oz. of boiling water

1 Tablespoon of fresh ginger (thinly sliced)

1 garlic clove (peeled and crushed)

2 lemons (juiced)

5 peppercorns, whole (if tolerated on AIP)

Directions:

1. First, you put water on the stove to boil.
2. After which you combine all ingredients in a strainer or teapot.
3. Then you pour boiling water into the pot and steep for 10 minutes.
4. Finally, you strain and enjoy!

Moroccan-Inspired Breakfast Skillet
Serves: 4 servings

Ingredients

2 tablespoons of solid cooking fat (coconut oil or lard work well here)

1 small bunch chard (with stems removed, separated, and both stems and leaves chopped)

1 teaspoon of ground turmeric

⅛ Teaspoon of cinnamon

½ cup of raisins

1 lb. of pastured ground pork

1 medium sweet potato, diced (about 2 cups)

3 cloves of garlic (minced)

½ teaspoon of sea salt

1 teaspoon of apple cider vinegar

Directions:

1. First, you place the ground pork in the bottom of a cold heavy-bottomed pan, and break up slightly with a utensil.
2. After which you turn on medium-high heat, and cook, stirring, until the meat is browned and has absorbed all of the fat (NOTE: don't drain it off!).
3. After that, you turn off the heat, transfer to a large bowl and set aside.
4. At this point, you place the same pan back on the stove, add the solid cooking fat, and turn the heat to medium-high.
5. Then when the fat has melted and the pan is hot, add the sweet potatoes and cook, stirring, for five minutes.
6. This is when you add the chard stems and cook for 3 more minutes.
7. Furthermore, you add the garlic, turmeric, sea salt, and cinnamon, and stir to combine.
8. After which you cook for a few more minutes, until the sweet potatoes are just soft.
9. Then you add the chard leaves, apple cider vinegar, and raisins to the pan.
10. After that, you continue cooking until chard has wilted, about a minute or two.
11. Finally, you turn off the heat, salt to taste, and serve warm

Kedgeree

Serves: 4

Ingredients

1¼ lb. cod, lingcod or better still other firm white fish, skin on

1 tablespoon of solid fat (such as coconut oil or lard)

½ teaspoon of turmeric powder

1 large cauliflower (divided into large florets)

2 tablespoons of finely chopped dill

Lemon wedges to serve

½ lb. of smoked sablefish (or better still smoked haddock, skin on)

1 bay leaf

1 onion (thinly sliced)

1 large cinnamon stick (snapped in half)

3 tablespoons of finely chopped curly parsley

Generous pinch of sea salt

Directions:

1. First, you put the fish skin side down into a large sauté pan with the bay leaf and cover with filtered water.
2. After which you bring up to a simmer and poach gently for about 5 minutes until just cooked.
3. After that, you remove the fish and bay leaf with a slotted spoon onto a large plate and set aside somewhere warm.
4. At this point, you pour the liquor through a sieve into a large jug and keep aside.
5. This is when you wipe out the pan.
6. Then you put the cauliflower florets into a food processor fitted with the "S" blade and pulse 4 or 5 short times until the caulis is slightly larger than plump grains of rice.
7. Furthermore, you heat the fat in the pan and add the onions.
8. After that you gently sweat them for about 6-8 minutes until soft and translucent.

9. Then you stir in the turmeric, cinnamon stick and reserved bay leaf and cook another minute or two.
10. At this point, you add the cauliflower and stir to combine with the onions and take on the turmeric color.
11. In addition, you add ½ cup of the poaching liquor and cook for around 5 minutes until it is just tender with a little bite to it still.
12. After which you remove the skins from the fish and break the flesh into large flakes.
13. Finally, you add this to the caulis and quickly warm through.
14. Then throw in the herbs, give a final stir and serve immediately with lemon wedges on the side.

Piña Colada Smoothie Bowl

Serves: 1 serving

Ingredients

1 small banana

2 scoops (20g) collagen hydrolysate

Pinch of sea salt

1½ cups of frozen pineapple chunks

½ - ⅔ cup coconut milk (depending on desired thickness)

2 teaspoons of lime juice

1 teaspoon of alcohol-free vanilla extracts

Additional pineapple chunks, unsweetened shredded coconut and lime zest (it optional for serving)

Directions:

1. First, you puree frozen pineapple, collagen, banana, coconut milk, lime juice, vanilla and sea salt in a high-powered blender until smooth.
2. After which you pour into an individual serving bowl or glass.
3. Then you garnish with additional pineapple chunks, shredded coconut and lime zest.
4. Make sure you serve cold.

Breakfast Risotto with Greens

Serves: 4

Ingredients

1 tablespoon of solid cooking fat (I prefer lard)

1 bunch rainbow chard, tough stems removed, leaves cut into long ribbons (about 5 cups)

1 teaspoon of dried oregano

¼ teaspoon of turmeric

1 pound of butternut squash, peeled and cubed (about 4 cups)

1 clove garlic (minced)

1 teaspoon of sea salt

½ teaspoon of onion powder

¼ teaspoon of cinnamon

Directions:

1. First, you place the squash in food processor and pulse for 30 seconds, until squash is "riced." (**Note:** Don't over process!)
2. After which you heat solid cooking fat in a large skillet on medium-low heat.
3. Then when fat has melted, add squash.
4. At this point, you cook, stirring occasionally, for 4-5 minutes.
5. This is when you add garlic, cook until fragrant.
6. Furthermore, you add remaining herbs, spices.
7. After that, you stir to incorporate, cook 4-5 more minutes.
8. Add chard and place lid over skillet for 2 minutes, allowing chard to wilt.
9. Then you remove lid, stir to combine wilted chard.
10. Finally, you remove from heat and serve.

Serves: 4 servings

Ingredients

¾ cup of finely shredded coconut

3 cups of coconut milk

Generous pinch of salt

Toasted coconut chips (optional for serving)

1 large head of cauliflower

2 tablespoons of coconut butter

Zest of a large lemon (you should save the juice for something else)

Spoonful softly whipped coconut cream (it optional for serving)

Handful mixed berries (it optional for serving)

Directions:

1. First, you cut the cauliflower into florets and put them into your food processor with the 'S' blade, not forgetting the stalks.
2. After which you pulse about 8-10 times until the caulis is the same consistency as large grains of rice (NOTE: you may need to do this in two batches).
3. Remember that pulsing puts you in control; if you simply press the 'on' button you risk ending up with purée!
4. After that, you transfer the riced cauliflower to a large pan, add the remaining porridge ingredients and stir to combine everything.
5. Then you bring up to a simmer, cover with a lid, and cook for about 25-30 minutes until the caulis is tender and the porridge nice and creamy.

IT IS OPTIONAL:

6. Furthermore, while the porridge is cooling, whip the coconut cream.
7. Then you start by removing your chilled coconut milk from the fridge, turning it upside down and opening it up with a can opener.
8. After that, you pour the thin coconut water into a jar and keep for another purpose, such as in smoothies.

9. Finally, you scoop out the cream and beat with a balloon whisk until soft peaks form, then transfer to a small container until needed.

Notes

Make sure you put a can of coconut milk in the fridge at least the night before you want to make whipped cream.

Prosciutto Meatloaf Muffins with Fig Jam
Serves: 12 muffins

Ingredients

2 lbs. of ground beef

5 oz. of AIP-friendly prosciutto

½ teaspoon of sea salt

2 cups of white sweet potato (cubed)

½ teaspoon of granulated garlic

1 tablespoon of thyme leaves

Directions:

1. Meanwhile, you heat oven to 350 degrees F.
2. After which you line 12 muffin cups with prosciutto slices ensuring the sides and bottom are covered.
3. After that, you set a steamer basket over a pot of boiling water.
4. At this point, you place sweet potatoes in the basket, cover, and let steam cook for about 10-12 minutes until the potatoes easily break apart with a fork.
5. This is when you place cooked sweet potatoes, thyme leaves, beef, and sea salt in a high powered blender or food processor.
6. Furthermore, you process until the sweet potatoes and meat are pureed into a paste.
7. After that, you spoon ⅓ cup of the meatloaf mixture into each prosciutto-lined muffin cup.
8. Then you bake on the middle rack of the oven for 23 minutes.
9. In addition, you spoon 1 tablespoon of Fig Jam on top of each muffin and broil on high for 2-3 minutes until the jam begins to caramelize.
10. Finally, you remove and serve warm with extra Fig Jam on the side.

Fig Jam
Serves: 1 cup

Ingredients

¼ cup of orange Juice

1 teaspoon of orange zest

Pinch sea salt

1 cup of dried black mission figs (with stems removed)

2 sprigs of thyme

¼ teaspoon of cinnamon

1 tablespoon of apple cider vinegar

Directions:

1. First, you place the dried figs, orange juice, thyme sprigs, and enough water to barely cover the figs in your smallest saucepan.
2. After which you bring to a boil, cover, and lower the heat to maintain a simmer for 20 minutes.
3. After that, you place figs, remaining water from the pot, and the rest of the Fig Jam ingredients in a blender or food processor.
4. Then you blend on low speed until a jam-like consistency has formed, about 30 seconds.

Italian-Spiced 50/50 Sausages

Serves: 8-10 patties

Ingredients

1 pound of pastured ground pork

1 tablespoon of minced fresh thyme

½ teaspoon of garlic powder

1 tablespoon of solid cooking fat (coconut oil, tallow, lard, or duck fat)

1 pound of grass-fed ground beef

1 tablespoon of minced fresh oregano

1 tablespoon of minced fresh parsley (it is optional)

½ teaspoon of sea salt

Directions:

1. First, you place the ground beef, herbs, pork, garlic powder and salt in a large bowl and combine well with your hands.
2. After which you form into 8-10 patties and place on a plate.
3. After that, you heat the solid cooking fat in the bottom of a cast-iron skillet or frying pan on medium heat.
4. At this point, when the fat is melted and the pan is hot, add patties, cook 10 minutes a side, or until thoroughly cooked (NOTE: you may have to do this in two batches).
5. Alternately, you can bake them at 400 degrees for about 20 minutes or until they are cooked throughout.

Variation: you should feel free to switch up the protein in these--you can make them 100% beef or pork, or add some lamb into the mix!

Christina's Turkey Breakfast Sausage

Serves: 4

Ingredients

2 teaspoons of fresh sage

1 teaspoon of fresh thyme

½ teaspoon of cinnamon

2 tablespoons of coconut oil

1 pound of ground turkey

1 teaspoon of fresh rosemary

½ teaspoon of garlic powder

1 teaspoon of sea salt

Directions:

1. First, you combine all ingredients except the oil and refrigerate for at least 30 minutes, overnight preferred.
2. After which you add the oil and shape into four patties.
3. After that, you cook in a lightly oiled skillet over medium heat, about five minutes per side or until no longer pink in the middle.
4. Alternatively, you bake at 400F for about 25 minutes.
5. Then you serve hot.

Three-Herb Beef Breakfast Patties

Serves: 6-8

Ingredients

1 tablespoon of fresh rosemary

1 tablespoon of fresh sage

1 tablespoon of coconut oil

2lbs grass-fed of ground beef

1 tablespoon of fresh thyme

1 teaspoon of sea salt

Directions:

1. First, you combine the ground beef, fresh herbs, and sea salt in a large bowl.
2. After which you form into patties using the palms of your hands.
3. After that, you heat some of the coconut oil in a cast-iron skillet on medium heat.
4. Then you cook the patties for about 5-8 minutes a side, until nicely browned on the outside and cooked throughout.

Spicy Roasted Sweet Potato & Pineapple Salad
Serves: 4 servings

Ingredients

1 tablespoon of lard or bacon fat (melted)

1 ¼ teaspoon of sea salt (divided)

2 tablespoons of lime juice

2 tablespoons of minced chives

2 pounds sweet potatoes (peeled and chopped into ½-inch cubes)

4 cups of diced pineapple (divided)

1-inch chunk ginger root (peeled and chopped)

¼ teaspoon of fish sauce

½ cup of cilantro leaves (chopped)

Directions:

1. Meanwhile, you heat oven to 400 degrees F. Line two baking sheets with parchment paper.
2. After which you toss sweet potatoes with lard and 1 teaspoon sea salt on one baking sheet.
3. After that, you spread 3 cups pineapple out onto second baking sheet.
4. Then you bake sweet potato and pineapple for about 40 to 45 minutes, tossing halfway through.
5. At this point, you remove from oven and let cool slightly while you make the dressing.
6. Furthermore, in a food processor, combine remaining ginger, 1 cup pineapple, remaining ¼ teaspoon sea salt, and ginger, lime, and fish sauce until smooth.
7. After that, you transfer sweet potatoes and pineapple to a serving bowl and toss with spicy pineapple dressing, cilantro, and chives.
8. Finally, you serve warm or at room temperature.

Shrimp Salad with Cilantro-Lime Ranch Dressing
Serves: 2

Ingredients

1 carrot (grated)

½ cup of Cilantro-Lime Ranch Dressing (recipe below)

½ head romaine (shredded)

1-2 tablespoons of cilantro (for garnish)

12 ounces peeled (deveined shrimp)

1 avocado (pitted and chopped into chunks)

½ green apple (cored and chopped into chunks)

1 tablespoon of coconut oil

Directions:

1. **First, you p**lace the coconut oil in the bottom of a skillet on medium heat.
2. At this point, when the fat has melted and the pan is hot, you sauté the shrimp in batches, making sure not to crowd, and cooking for 1-2 minutes or until opaque and fully cooked.
3. After that, you remove and set aside to cool.
4. **After which you p**lace the romaine, grated carrot, green apple, avocado, and cilantro in a large bowl with the shrimp.
5. Then you arrange, or toss to combine.
6. Finally, you serve with cilantro-lime ranch dressing.

Cilantro-Lime Ranch Dressing

Serves: 1 cup

Ingredients

¼ cup of extra-virgin olive oil

1 lime (juiced)

1 clove of garlic

1 tablespoon of fresh cilantro

⅓ Cup of coconut concentrate

½ cup of filtered water

1 teaspoon of apple cider vinegar

½ teaspoon of sea salt

Directions:

1. First, you place all ingredients except for the cilantro in a blender and mix until thoroughly combined (**NOTE:** if the dressing is too thick, thin with water until the desired consistency is reached).
2. After which you add the cilantro and blend for 10 seconds more, or until just combined.

Notes

Note: Remember that in order to measure the concentrate, it is best to soften it in a warm water bath before use as it is solid at room temperature.

However, coconut concentrate is otherwise known as "coconut butter" or "coconut manna" and is solid at room temperature. It is not the cream at the top of a can of coconut milk!

Ginger-Lime Salmon with Watermelon Mint Salsa
Serves: 2 servings

Ingredients

1 tablespoon of olive oil

1 teaspoon of grated fresh ginger

Arugula for serving

2 6-oz wild salmon filets (With skin on)

1 tablespoon of lime juice

1 teaspoon of apple cider vinegar

¼ teaspoon of sea salt

Directions:

1. First, you pat salmon filets dry and lay flat, skin side down, in a shallow glass dish.
2. After which you whisk together olive oil, lime juice, ginger, vinegar, and sea salt in a small glass bowl.
3. After that, you pour marinade evenly over the salmon filets.
4. Then you allow salmon to marinade for about 25-30 minutes.
5. In the meantime, preheat broiler to 425 degrees F.
6. At this point, you arrange an oven rack 6-8 inches away from the oven broiler element.
7. This is when you transfer salmon to an oven-safe rimmed baking sheet.
8. Furthermore, you broil for 5-7 minutes, depending on the thickness of the salmon filet; until the salmon is cooked through for well-done salmon or until the center is a medium pink for medium-done salmon.
9. Then you serve a top arugula with the Watermelon Mint Salsa (below).

Watermelon Mint Salsa
Serves: 1½ cups

Ingredients

2 tablespoons of lime juice

½ teaspoon of grated fresh ginger

1 ½ cups of diced seedless watermelon

1 tablespoon of sliced fresh mint leaves

1 tablespoon of olive oil

2 teaspoons of red wine vinegar or balsamic vinegar

¼ teaspoon of sea salt

2 tablespoons of sliced fresh cilantro leaves

Directions:

1. First, you whisk together the olive oil, lime, vinegar of choice, ginger, and sea salt.
2. After which you toss with the watermelon in a medium size bowl.
3. Then you mix in the fresh herbs.

Carrot, Cucumber, and Avocado Salad
Serves: 4

Ingredients

2 tablespoons of honey

1 teaspoon of sea salt

1 lb. rainbow carrots (halved lengthwise and cut into 3-inch chunks)

Olive oil (to taste)

¼ cup of apple cider vinegar

1 lb. pickling cucumbers (thinly sliced with a mandolin)

½-inch piece of ginger (finely grated)

1 bunch cilantro (chopped)

1 avocado (cubed)

Directions:

1. First, you place the cider vinegar and honey in a small bowl and whisk until combined.
2. After which you pour over the cucumber slices, sprinkle with sea salt and ginger, and stir to combine.
3. After that, you place in the refrigerator for at least 2 hours or overnight.
4. Then when you are ready to make the salad, bring a large pot of water to a boil on the stovetop.
5. At this point, you blanch the carrots for about 3-4 minutes, and then drain and rinse with cold water.
6. This is when you strain the cucumber mixture, reserving some of the juice to add back to the salad.
7. In addition, you add the cilantro, avocado, carrots, and cucumber mixture to a large bowl and toss to combine.
8. Finally, you add back some of the cucumber juice and olive oil to taste and serve.

Notes

Note:

Remember that this recipe doesn't keep well once mixed, so if you'd like to serve it for multiple meals make sure you keep the cucumber mixture separate and cut the avocados fresh!

Bistro Chicken Salad with Garlic-Thyme Vinaigrette

Ingredients

1 ½ pounds of chicken breast

1 teaspoon of garlic powder

2 tablespoons of balsamic vinegar

1 teaspoon of minced garlic

6 slices of bacon

2 teaspoons of dried thyme

1 teaspoon of fine sea salt

1 large head red leaf lettuce (torn into 1-inch pieces)

1 large shallot (thinly sliced)

Optional: freshly grated carrots and sliced avocado

Garlic-Thyme Vinaigrette **(below)**

Directions:

1. First, in a large cast iron skillet, you cook bacon until crispy on both sides over medium heat.
2. After which you transfer cooked bacon to a cutting board and dice with a sharp knife.
3. After that, you leave the rendered bacon fat in the skillet.
4. Then you set chopped bacon aside.
5. At this point, you pat the chicken breasts dry.
6. Furthermore, you mix together the thyme; garlic powder and sea salt and rub on all sides of the chicken breasts.
7. After that, you cook the chicken in the bacon fat over medium heat until golden on both sides, about 3 to 5 minutes per side, until slightly pink in the center.
8. After which you transfer the chicken breasts to a large cutting board and slice into ½-inch thick slices.
9. This is when you return chicken to the skillet and finish cooking for 5 minutes until cooked through and juicy.
10. In addition, you sprinkle the balsamic vinegar over the chicken and toss until coated.
11. Then arrange the salad by layering the lettuce, warm chicken, shallot, garlic, bacon, and optional carrots and avocado.
12. Finally, you drizzle with Garlic-Thyme Dressing.

Zesty Detox Salad
Serves: 4

Ingredients

1 bunch watercress, chopped (about 1 cup tightly packed)

2 small or betterstill1 large head of broccoli (finely chopped)

¾ cup of olive oil

2 anchovy fillets

1 avocado (cubed)

1 bunch cilantro, chopped (about 1 cup tightly packed)

2 cups of microgreens (about 3 ounces)

2 small of 1 large beet (cut into ½-inch cubes)

½ lemons (juiced)

1 clove of garlic

Directions:

1. First, you combine the cilantro, microgreens, watercress, broccoli, and beets in a large bowl and toss to combine.
2. After which you place the olive oil, lemon juice, anchovies, and garlic in a blender and blend for 30 seconds or until fully combined.
3. Then you toss the dressing with the salad and add the avocado.

Note: If you are preparing this salad for later, I suggest you keep the greens and dressing separate and add avocado fresh.

You can keeps for 1 to 2 days in the refrigerator.

Mediterranean Cauliflower Couscous Salad

Serves: 4 servings

Ingredients

3½ cups of uncooked rice cauliflower

¾ cup of peeled, seeded, and diced cucumber

½ cup of dried cranberries

⅓ Cup of diced red onion

1 tablespoon of minced fresh dill

1 tablespoon of olive oil

¼ teaspoon of sea salt

⅔ Cup of finely chopped parsley (loosely packed)

⅓ Cup of diced dried Turkish figs

4 green onions (sliced crosswise)

Vinaigrette:

1 tablespoon + ½ teaspoon of lemon juice

½ teaspoon of grated orange zest

¼ teaspoon of dried dill

3 tablespoons of olive oil

1 tablespoon of apple cider vinegar

½ teaspoon of sea salt

¼ teaspoon of garlic powder

Directions:

1. First, you heat olive oil in a large stainless steel pan over medium heat.
2. After which you add rice cauliflower to the pan and season with sea salt.
3. After that, you sauté for 5 minutes, tossing only every 2 minutes to prevent sticking, until lightly browned and tender (Note: ensure you do not overcook the rice or it will be mushy).

4. At this point, you set the cooked cauliflower rice aside to cool completely.

NOTE: you may do this by leaving it at room temperature for about 30 minutes or by scooping onto a plate and placing in the refrigerator until cooled.

5. In the meantime, you combine the remaining salad ingredients in a serving bowl.
6. This is when you toss in the cooled and cooked rice cauliflower.
7. Then you make the vinaigrette by whisking all of its ingredients together in a small bowl.
8. Finally, you toss gently with the salad until evenly incorporated.

Thai-Inspired Pork Salad

Serves: 2 servings

Ingredients

1 lb. of ground pork

2 large cloves garlic (peeled and thinly sliced)

Zest and juice of one large lime

1 tablespoon of fish sauce

½ packed cup cilantro leaves (chopped)

Extra lime wedges (to serve)

1 teaspoon of lard (or better still other solid fat)

1 1/2-inch piece ginger (peeled and finely grated)

5 shallots (peeled and thinly sliced)

4 green onions (thinly sliced on the diagonal)

1 tablespoon of coconut aminos

½ packed of cup Thai basil leaves (chopped)

¼ packed cup mint leaves (chopped)

Directions:

1. First, you heat the fat on a fairly high heat in a large skillet or wok and tip in the pork.
2. After which you cook for about 4-5 minutes until the liquid has all but evaporated and the pork is beginning to brown.
3. Then whilst this is happening, break down the ground meat's tendency to clump with a long handled wooden fork or spoon.
4. After that, you add the ginger, garlic and shallots and cook for 3 minutes, stirring very frequently.

NOTE: if you want the pork to crisp up but not burn on the bottom of the pan, I suggest you keep that fork/spoon moving.

5. At this point, you stir in the lime zest and juice, together with the green onions, and cook a further minute.

6. Furthermore, you tip in the fish sauce and coconut aminos and cook one minute more, scraping the sediment off the bottom of the pan all the while.
7. Finally, you remove from the heat, throw in the herbs, give it all a good mix and serve with a decent wedge of lime on the side.

Notes

Delicious hot, warm or cold – I suggest you served with kelp noodles or in lettuce boats. With noodles included, this recipe serves three.

Summer Grapefruit Salad
Serves: 4

Ingredients

1 kiwi

¼ cup of lemon juice

1 tablespoon of chopped chives

1 pink grapefruit

1 avocado

Pinch of sea salt

1 small head bib lettuce

Dressing:

Pinch of salt

2 tablespoons of extra virgin olive oil

1 tablespoon of apple cider vinegar

Directions:

1. First, you peel the skin from the grapefruit with a sharp knife, making sure you remove all the white.
2. After which you cut up the flesh into small ½-inch cubes; set aside.
3. After that, you peel the skin from the kiwi and slice thinly with a sharp knife; set aside.
4. Then you peel the avocado, remove the pit and cut into small cubes.
5. Furthermore, in a small dish, you cover the avocado with lemon juice and a pinch of salt, and let marinate for a few minutes.
6. In the meantime, cut your bib lettuce into small, bite-sized pieces.
7. At this point, you place all ingredients in a large bowl and mix delicately (NOTE: Really use light hands here!)
8. This is when you drizzle the dressing on the salad and sprinkle chives for garnish.
9. Then serve immediately.

Purslane with Crispy Bacon and Blueberries

Serves: 2 as a main, 4 as a side

Ingredients

For the salad:

½ lb. of purslane (larger stalks removed)

1 large avocado (chopped)

8 slices of bacon

¾ cup of blueberries

3 oz. of radishes (thinly sliced)

Ingredients for the dressing:

1 tablespoon of lemon juice

Good pinch of sea salt

1 tablespoon of golden balsamic vinegar

2 tablespoons of olive oil

Directions:

1. First, you put the bacon slices onto a large baking tray and broil for 8 mins or so until nice and crispy.
2. After which you transfer onto a plate lined with absorbent kitchen paper and allow cooling and hardening.
3. After that, you put the other salad ingredients into a large bowl.
4. Then you crunch the bacon slices between your finger tips and allow the crispy shards to fall over the salad.
5. Finally, you whisk the dressing ingredients together, add to the salad and toss well.

Shrimp Ceviche Salad
Serves: 2 servings

Ingredients

1 ½ cups of chopped green apple

1 cup of chopped cooked shrimp

2 tablespoons of finely chopped mint

2 tablespoons of lemon juice

¼ teaspoon of garlic powder

1 ½ cups of seeded and chopped cucumber

Meat of 1 avocado (diced)

¼ cup of finely chopped parsley

½ teaspoon of sea salt

2 tablespoons of olive oil

Directions:

1. First, you mix all ingredients together in a serving bowl.
2. After which you refrigerate for at least two hours to let flavors marry.
3. Then you stir well before serving.

Serves: 2 servings

Ingredients

½ cup of carrots (shredded)

2 tablespoons of chopped green onion

½ tablespoon of extra virgin olive oil

½ teaspoon of ground turmeric

¼ teaspoon of sea salt

1 small head of broccoli (chopped)

⅓ Cup of coconut cream

½ tablespoon of apple cider vinegar

¾ teaspoon of ground ginger

¼ teaspoon of ground cinnamon

Directions:

First, you combine all ingredients in a large bowl and refrigerate at least 30 minutes to let the flavors meld before serving.

Rib boned Asparagus and Fennel Salad

Serves: 2

Ingredients

1 large fennel bulb

1 lemon (juiced)

¼ teaspoon of sea salt

1-2 pounds asparagus (with white ends trimmed)

¼ cup of extra-virgin olive oil

¼ teaspoon of lemon zest

Directions:

1. First, you take the asparagus and use a vegetable peeler to create long "ribbons" and place them in a bowl.
2. Note: I find it easiest to start towards the spear end, and then come back and do the bottoms. Remember that you will end up with a little "core" at the end; you can either slice this thin with a knife and add to the salad or discard.
3. After which you use a mandolin slicer on the thinnest setting to slice the fennel bulb.
4. Then you add it to the bowl with the asparagus.
5. Finally, you add the olive oil, lemon juice, zest, and sea salt to the asparagus and fennel.
6. At this point, you toss to combine.

Honey-Lime Chicken & Strawberry Salad
Serves: 2

Ingredients

1 tablespoon of coconut oil

1 tablespoon of honey

2 tablespoons of mint (sliced)

½ cucumber (peeled and chopped)

Sea salt

1 lb. of chicken breast (cut into ¾-inch pieces)

½ limes (juiced)

6 strawberries (sliced)

½ avocado (diced)

4 cups of romaine lettuce (shredded)

Directions:

1. First, you heat coconut oil in a skillet over medium high heat.
2. After which you add chopped chicken breast, sprinkle with sea salt, and let cook undisturbed until golden brown for 3 minutes.
3. After that, you flip chicken, sprinkle with more salt and continue to cook for about 2 more minutes.
4. At this point, you add lime juice and honey to pan.
5. Then you stir to coat chicken.
6. Furthermore, you turn heat to medium, cover skillet with a lid, and let the chicken finish cooking for 2 to 3 more minutes.
7. After that, you stir to coat the chicken in the honey-lime glaze and set aside to cool while you prepare the salad.
8. This is when you divide the remaining salad ingredients between two plates. Top with chicken and drizzle with two tablespoons Strawberry-Lime Dressing (recipe below).

Early Spring Salad with Grapefruit and Ginger Vinaigrette

Serves: 4

Ingredients

1 lemon (juiced)

¼ teaspoon of ginger powder

4 cups of arugula

1 fennel bulb, sliced thinly with a mandolin or better still sharp knife

¼ cup of extra-virgin olive oil

1 tablespoon of apple cider vinegar

¼ teaspoon of sea salt

1 large or better still 2 small grapefruits (peeled and sectioned)

Directions:

1. First, you place the olive oil, apple cider vinegar, lemon juice, ginger powder, and sea salt in a small bowl and whisk to combine; set aside.
2. After which you place the arugula, grapefruit sections, and fennel slices in a large bowl.
3. Then you toss with the dressing just before serving.

Note: If your grapefruit is particularly large, I suggest you may want to slice the sections in half or serve with a knife.

Storage: you can keep for a couple of days separated in the refrigerator--toss fresh with dressing before serving.

Simple Beet and Fennel Salad

Serves: 3-4

Ingredients

For the dressing:

1 tablespoon of apple cider vinegar

¼ teaspoon of sea salt

½ cup of olive oil

½ lemons (juiced)

1 garlic clove (minced)

Ingredients For the salad:

1 cucumber

Sprig of mint (chopped)

4 beets (tops removed)

1 fennel bulb

Handful of parsley (chopped)

Directions:

1. First, you place all of the dressing ingredients in a small bowl and whisk to combine; set aside.
2. After which you slice the beets, cucumber, and fennel on the thinnest setting with a mandolin or very carefully with a knife.
3. After that, you place in a large bowl and toss with the dressing.

Fig and Arugula Salad with Raspberry Vinaigrette

Serves: 6

Ingredients

½ cup of fresh raspberries

2 tablespoons of unsweetened coconut flakes (it is optional)

8 dried figs (sliced thinly)

½ cup of olive oil

2 tablespoons of apple-cider vinegar

¼ teaspoon of sea salt

6 ounces arugula

Directions:

1. First, you place the olive oil, raspberries, apple-cider vinegar, shredded coconut and sea salt in a blender and blend on high for a few minutes until the dressing has a creamy texture, stopping to give the motor breaks (NOTE: you won't have to blend nearly as long if you are not using the coconut).
2. After which you place the arugula and figs in a large bowl, add dressing and toss.

Jane's Mango and Coconut Summer Salad

Serves: 4

Ingredients

Ingredients for the Salad:

2 small mangoes (cut into 1-inch pieces)

1-2 avocadoes (cut into large chunks)

4 cups of mixed greens

½ cup of thick coconut flakes

½ cucumbers (chopped)

Ingredients for the Cinnamon-Lime Dressing:

1 lime (juiced)

¼ teaspoon of sea salt

⅛ Teaspoon of ginger powder

¼ cup of extra-virgin olive oil

1 tablespoon of apple-cider vinegar

⅛ Teaspoon of cinnamon

Directions:

1. First, you place all of the salad ingredients in a large bowl except for the coconut chips and avocado.
2. After which you place all of the ingredients for the dressing in a small bowl and whisk to combine.
3. After that, you add to the salad and toss to combine.
4. Then you garnish with coconut flakes and avocado chunks.

Pomegranate and Arugula Salad with Fennel and Blood-Orange Vinaigrette

Serves: 4

Ingredients

Ingredients for the Blood-Orange Vinaigrette:

1/2 cup of extra-virgin olive oil

1/4 teaspoon of ginger powder

2 blood oranges (juiced)

2 teaspoons of Ume plum vinegar

Ingredients for the Salad:

1 cup of pomegranate seeds

4 cups of baby arugula

1 small fennel bulb (sliced thinly)

Directions:

1. First, you combine the orange juice, olive oil, Ume plum vinegar, ginger powder, and sea salt in a small bowl and whisk to incorporate; set aside.
2. After which you combine the arugula, fennel slices, and pomegranate seeds in a bowl.
3. Then you toss with the blood-orange vinaigrette and serve immediately.

Summer Cabbage and Jicama Coleslaw

Serves: 6-8

Ingredients

For the dressing:

½ cup of warm filtered water

2 tablespoons of apple-cider vinegar

¼ teaspoon of salt

½ cup of coconut concentrate (warmed in a bowl of hot water)

⅓ Cup of extra-virgin olive oil

½ lemons (juiced)

3-4 cloves of raw garlic

Ingredients For the salad:

½ head green cabbage (shredded)

½ red onions (sliced thinly)

1 handful of parsley (finely chopped)

½ head of purple cabbage (shredded)

Salt (to taste)

½ pound jicama (peeled and sliced thinly)

Directions:

1. First, you place the coconut concentrate, warm water, olive oil, garlic cloves and salt in a blender and blend on high for a minute or two, until the sauce thickens.

NOTE: if it is too thick, add warm water a tablespoon at a time until it reaches the desired consistency; set aside.

2. After which you place the cabbage in a large bowl and lightly sprinkle with salt.
3. After that, you massage cabbage for a few minutes with your hands, until some of the tough fibers break down a little bit.
4. Then you add the red onion, jicama, and parsley and toss with dressing.

5. Finally, you serve immediately (**NOTE:** if you store leftovers in the fridge, be forewarned that the dressing hardens a bit and you might want to bring back to room temperature before serving).

Garlic "Mayo"

Make sure you cool for an hour at room temperature or 20 minutes in the refrigerator.

Serves: 1½ cups

Ingredients

½ cup of warm filtered water

¼ teaspoon of salt

½ cup of coconut concentrate (warmed in a bowl of hot water)

¼ cup of extra-virgin olive oil

3-4 cloves garlic

Directions:

1. First, you place the coconut concentrate, warm water, olive oil, garlic cloves and salt in a blender and blend on high for a minute or two, until the sauce thickens.
2. After which you let cool for an hour at room temperature – alternately, you can place it in the refrigerator for 20 minutes.

NOTE: if you would like to use the sauce in a cold dish, I suggest you thin with water until the desired consistency are reached.

You can store well in the refrigerator, but hardens.

Let come to room-temperature or warm gently before using.

Curried Chicken Salad

Serves: 4

Ingredients

1 teaspoon of apple-cider vinegar

2 teaspoons of powdered turmeric

¼ teaspoon of sea salt

¼ cup of red onion (chopped)

2 tablespoons of parsley (chopped)

½ cup of garlic "mayo", room-temperature or better still slightly warm

½ lemons (juiced)

1 teaspoon of powdered ginger

1 lb. of pastured chicken breast (cooked and shredded)

¼ cup of raisins (it is optional)

Directions:

1. First, you combine the mayo, lemon juice, apple-cider vinaigrette, turmeric, ginger, and sea salt in a bowl and whisk to combine.
2. After which you add the chicken breast, red onion, and raisins and stir.
3. Then you serve garnished with chopped parsley.

Cabbage and Avocado Salad with Blood Orange Vinaigrette

Serves: 6

Ingredients

1 small red onion (thinly sliced)

1 handful parsley (chopped)

4 tablespoons of olive oil

1 or 2 avocados (cubed)

1 head savoy cabbage (shredded)

3 carrots (grated)

2 blood oranges (juiced)

2 teaspoons of coconut vinegar

3 teaspoons of salt

Directions:

1. First, you combine cabbage, onion, carrots, and most of the parsley.
2. After which you combine the juice from the oranges, olive oil, coconut vinegar, and salt in a small bowl.
3. Then you toss the dressing with the cabbage mixture, adding avocado and parsley on the top.

Winter Kale Salad
Serves: 4

Ingredients

3 tablespoon of olive oil

¼ cup of red onion (minced)

Sea salt (to taste)

2 large bunches of kale (to me variety doesn't matter – I like to mix a couple different types)

2 carrots (grated)

½ cucumber (chopped)

Juice of 1 lemon

Directions:

1. First, you wash, stem and chop the kale.
2. After which you place in a large bowl, add the olive oil and a pinch of salt.
3. After that, you massage the kale for 5-10 minutes or until the tough fibers begin to break down.
4. Remember that some varieties of kale are tougher than others and really need to be worked a bit.
5. At this point, when you are done with the kale will have considerably reduced in volume.
6. Finally, you combine with the grated carrots, cucumber, red onion, lemon juice, and more salt to taste if you wish.

Spinach Salad with Orange-Avocado Dressing

Serves: 4

Ingredients

Ingredients For the salad:

2 carrots (grated)

½ cucumber (chopped)

1 large bunch spinach (washed and stemmed)

10 Kalamata olives (halved)

Ingredient For the dressing:

1 orange (juiced)

¼ cup of apple-cider vinegar

½ teaspoon of salt

1 avocado

¼ cup of olive oil

¼ cup of water

½" piece of ginger (peeled and chopped)

Directions:

1. First, you wash and prepare the vegetables for the salad and place them in a large bowl.
2. After which you place all of the ingredients for the dressing into a blender and blend until incorporated.

NOTE: if the dressing is too thick, I suggest you keep adding water until it is the desired consistency.

3. Then you add some to the salad and toss, keeping the remainder in the refrigerator for another use.

Jicama, Pear, and Mint Salad with Citrus-Ginger Dressing

Serves: 4

Ingredients

2 small pears (sliced thinly)

2 tablespoons of olive oil

¼ teaspoon of ginger powder

1 lb. of jicama (sliced into matchsticks)

1 orange (juiced)

1 tablespoon of apple-cider vinegar

¼ teaspoon of sea salt

A few sprigs of mint and/or better still parsley

Directions:

1. First, you combine the jicama and pears in a bowl and set aside.
2. After which you combine the orange juice, cider vinegar, olive oil, ginger powder, and sea salt together in a small bowl.
3. Then you add to the jicama and pears and toss with the mint and parsley.

Radish and Jicama Tabbouli

Serves: 2 as a meal, 4 as a side

Ingredients

1 bunch radishes (finely chopped)

2 carrots (finely chopped)

8 Kalamata olives (minced)

¼ cup of olive oil

Salt to taste

1 bunch parsley (chopped)

½ lb. jicama (peeled and finely chopped)

1 cucumber (finely chopped)

1 tablespoon of mint (minced)

2 tablespoons of apple-cider vinegar

½ lemons (juiced)

Directions:

1. First, you combine all of the chopped veggies (parsley, radishes, jicama, carrots, cucumber, olives, and mint) in a large bowl.
2. After which you toss with the olive oil, cider vinegar, lemon, and salt.

Dessert

Cherry Carob Cookies

Serves: 12

Ingredients

¼ cup of carob powder

¾ teaspoon of baking soda

½ cup of palm shortening

¼ cup of coconut sugar

½ cup of dried cherries (chopped)

¾ cup of cassava flour

1 tablespoon + 1 teaspoon of gelatin

¾ teaspoon of sea salt

¼ cup of maple syrup

1 teaspoon of pure vanilla extract

Directions:

1. Meanwhile, you heat oven to 350 degrees F.
2. After which you line a baking sheet with parchment paper and set aside.
3. After that, you mix flour, carob, gelatin, baking soda and salt in a mixing bowl.
4. Then cream shortening, coconut sugar, maple, and vanilla together in another mixing bowl.
5. At this point, you place a fine mesh sieve over the shortening mixture bowl and sift the dry flour mixture into it.
6. This is when you carefully combine the flour mixture with the shortening mixture until a dough forms.
7. Furthermore, you add the cherries.
8. After that, you place in refrigerator for 10 minutes to chill.
9. In addition, you use approximately 1-2 tablespoon-sized scoops to place dough onto baking sheet, gently pressing down on each.
10. Finally, you bake for 9 minutes, and then begin checking every 2 minutes until they reach desired firmness (they will get firmer as they cool, so do not over bake).

Orange Blossom Panna Cotta with Rhubarb Compote

Serves: 4

Ingredients

For the panna cotta:

1 tablespoon of gelatin

2½ teaspoons of orange blossom water

2 tablespoons of orange blossom honey

Juice of 2-3 large sweet oranges, such as Cara Cara (to yield ¾ cup)

2¼ cups of full-fat coconut milk

Pinch of fine sea salt

Ingredient For the compote:

2 tablespoons of orange juice

1 teaspoon of orange blossom water

2 tablespoons of honey

1 lb. of thin rhubarb stems (cut down the middle if necessary), cut into 1½-inch pieces

Directions:

1. First you put ½ cup of the orange juice into a small pan, sprinkle over the gelatin and set aside for 5 minutes or so, until softened and spongy.
2. In the meantime, you put the remaining orange juice into a large jug, together with the coconut milk, orange blossom water and salt.
3. At this point, you heat the gelatin very gently until fully dissolved (NOTE: This process takes only seconds).
4. Furthermore, you stir in the honey, then remove from the heat and whisk the gelatin mixture into the coconut milk.
5. After which you divide the mixture between four glasses and put into the refrigerator to set (NOTE: Takes 3-4 hours).
6. In the meantime make the compote.
7. After that, you put the honey, orange juice and ¼ cup of filtered water into a sauté pan and bring up to a simmer.
8. Then you add the rhubarb, preferably in one layer, cover with a lid, then turn the heat down and cook gently for 4-5 minutes until tender but still retaining its shape.

9. Furthermore, you remove the rhubarb from the pan with a slotted spoon and set aside.
10. This is when you reduce the liquid by half, stir in the orange blossom water and pour over the rhubarb.
11. This is the point you leave to cool completely.
12. Finally, if you want to serve, put spoonfuls of the compote on top of the panna cotta just before eating.

Pear & Plum Cranberry Crumble

Serves: 4 servings

Ingredients

2 large D'anjou pears (cored and sliced into ⅓-inch slices)

5 ripe black plums (pitted and sliced into ½-inch slices)

¼ teaspoon of fine sea salt

½ teaspoon of cinnamon

1 tablespoon of lemon juice

2 tablespoons of coconut oil or lard

Crumble:

3 tablespoons of coconut flour

½ teaspoon of lemon zest

1 ¾ cups of sweet plantain chips

1 cup of dried unsweetened cranberries

2 tablespoons of melted coconut oil

Pinch of sea salt

Directions:

1. Meanwhile, you heat the oven to a 400 degree F broil.
2. After which you ensure the top rack is at least 6 inches from the heating element.
3. After that, in a 10- or 12-inch cast iron skillet, heat the coconut oil or lard over medium heat.
4. Then you add the sliced pears to the skillet and toss with the lemon juice.
5. At this point, you cook until medium-soft, about 5 minutes, stirring every couple of minutes.
6. Furthermore, you add the plums, cinnamon and sea salt to the skillet.
7. After that, you cook for 10 more minutes, continuing to stir every couple of minutes, until the fruit is softened and has released thick juices.
8. In the meantime, you make the crumble.

9. In addition, you combine the cranberries, coconut flour, and coconut oil in a food processor, for 15 seconds until the cranberries are sticky and have a medium-coarse texture.
10. This is when you add the lemon zest, sea salt and plantain chips and process for an additional 10 to 15 seconds until the chips are finely crumbled and combined with the cranberries.
11. After which you sprinkle the crumble topping into an even layer on the fruit.
12. Then you broil for 60 to 90 seconds until the crumble is golden being cautious not to burn it.
13. Finally, you remove from the oven and let cool 5 to 10 minutes before serving in individual dishes with a scoop of coconut whipped cream or ice cream, if desired.

Strawberry Ginger Ice Cream

Ingredients

1½ cups of coconut milk

Generous pinch of salt

¾ lb. of ripe strawberries (hulled)

¼ cup of raw honey

1½ teaspoons of ground ginger

Directions:

1. First, you place your ice cream container into the freezer to cool.
2. After which you put all the ingredients into a blender and blitz till smooth.
3. After that, you put into the fridge to chill, two hours or more.
4. At this point, you pour into an ice cream maker and churn, following the instructions in your manual.
5. Then you transfer the ice cream to your chilled container and put into the freezer to firm up.

NOTE: if you don't have a machine, I suggest you put the mixture into a freeze proof container and freeze till nearly firm.

6. Furthermore, you beat with a whisk until smooth again and return to the freezer.
7. In addition, you repeat two or three times and then leave to freeze.

NOTE: freezing in this manner results in larger ice crystals and a less creamy texture, but it will still be utterly delicious.

Serves: 4 cups

Ingredients

2 capsules of probiotics (any non-soil strain will do)

⅓ Cup of honey

4 cups of coconut cream (scooped from the top of 4 cans of coconut milk)

Directions:

1. First, you divide the coconut cream and probiotic powder evenly between each of your jars and mix well, and then cap the jars.
2. After which you place in a yogurt maker or instant Pot with yogurt setting and follow the manufacturer's instructions for yogurt. (In the instant pot, this takes about 12 hours).
3. After that, you refrigerate until cool.
4. Finally, you stir the honey into the yogurt and then run through an ice cream maker according to the manufacturer's instructions.

Notes:

You should refrigerate coconut milk overnight to ensure thick cream

Summer Fruit Gazpacho

Serves: 6

Ingredients

Ingredients For the gazpacho:

2 lbs. of strawberries

½ medium watermelon (approx. 10 inches across)

Ingredients For the raspberry sauce:

1 tablespoon of lemon juice

4 tablespoons of full fat coconut milk (from a can)

6 oz. of raspberries

Zest of one organic lemon

Mint leaves and some coconut milk for garnish

Directions:

1. First, you scoop out all the pulp from the watermelon with a spoon and place in a large pot.
2. After which you keep the skin of the watermelon and save in the refrigerator for later.
3. After that, you stem and quarter the strawberries.
4. At this point, you add to the watermelon.
5. Then with a hand-held mixer, mix the watermelon and strawberries until you obtain a smooth cream; set aside.
6. Furthermore, in a small bowl, mash the raspberries with a fork.
7. After that, you add the lemon juice, lemon zest, and coconut milk.
8. Then you mix well.

Direction on how to serve:

Remember that this gazpacho is best served chilled.

NOTE: if you prepare in advance, keep the soup and raspberry sauce in the refrigerator until it is time to serve. And for a pretty presentation, I suggest you serve the gazpacho in the skin of the watermelon! For each person, I will suggest you pour 2 ladles of gazpacho in a soup dish, drop a portion of raspberry sauce in the middle, and decorate with a few mint leaves and a drizzle of coconut milk.

Orange & Rose Honey Cake
Serves: 8 slices

Ingredients

2 green plantains (peeled and chopped)

¼ cup of liquid honey

2 tablespoons of orange blossom water

2 tablespoons of gelatin

¾ cup of cassava flour

½ teaspoon of baking soda

Honey, for drizzling

Coconut oil (for greasing pan)

½ cup of palm shortening (room temperature)

¼ cup of orange juice

1 tablespoon of rose water

⅓ Cup of hot water

½ teaspoon of cinnamon

¼ teaspoon of sea salt

1 cup of coconut flakes

1 lb. peeled = 1 lb, 12 oz unpeeled = 2 large green plantains

Directions:

1. Meanwhile, you heat oven to 350 degrees F.
2. After which you grease a 9-inch cake pan lightly with coconut oil.
3. After that, you puree coconut oil, green plantains palm, honey, orange juice and orange blossom water together in a blender until smooth.
4. Furthermore, in a small bowl, whisk together the gelatin and hot water until frothy.
5. After which you add to the blender.
6. Then in another small bowl, whisk together the cassava, cinnamon, baking soda, and sea salt.
7. In addition, you add to the blender and process until just combined.

8. At this point, you pour into prepared pan and smooth with the back of a spoon.
9. This is when you press coconut flakes into the top of the batter until evenly covered.
10. Finally, you bake for about 38-40 minutes until the edges have pulled away from the pan and the top of the coconut flakes are golden brown.
11. Then let cool for at least 15 minutes before slicing.
12. Remember that honey cake is best served warm.

Stuffed Pineapple
Serves: 8 servings

Ingredients

2 bananas (sliced)

½ cup of shredded unsweetened coconut

1 large pineapple (halved lengthwise)

½ cup of coconut milk

¼ teaspoon of ground cinnamon

Directions:

1. Meanwhile, you heat the oven to 325 degrees F.
2. After which with a melon baller, core the pineapple halves and then scoop the flesh out of the skin to make boats.
3. After that, you discard the core, and then divide the edible flesh evenly between the two pineapple halves.
4. Then you top with one of the sliced bananas and toss to combine with the pineapple.
5. At this point, you lay the pineapple boats, cut side up, on a baking sheet.
6. This is when you puree the remaining banana with the coconut milk and cinnamon in a blender, then pour into the pineapples, dividing equally.
7. Furthermore, you sprinkle the shredded coconut on top.
8. After that, you bake for 20-25 minutes or until golden brown on top.
9. Then you serve warm.

Raw Coconut Macaroons with "Chocolate" Ganache

Serves: 20

Ingredients

Ingredients for the macaroons:

1 tablespoon of coconut oil

2 tablespoons of alcohol-free vanilla extract

2 cups of shredded coconut

⅓ Cup of coconut cream (scooped from the top of a refrigerated can of coconut milk)

3 tablespoons of maple syrup

½ tablespoon of gelatin

"Chocolate" ganache:

2 tablespoons of carob powder

⅓ Cup of coconut milk

2 tablespoons of maple syrup

Directions:

1. First, in a pan on medium heat, mix together the coconut cream, coconut oil, maple syrup, and vanilla extract.
2. After which you remove from the heat and add the gelatin.
3. After that, you mix well with a whisk, making sure there is no clump.
4. Then you immediately add the shredded coconut and mix well again.
5. At this point, you line a baking sheet with parchment paper.
6. Furthermore, using a tablespoon to scoop out small portions of the coconut mixture to form little mounds, line the macaroons on the parchment paper (NOTE: eave a 1-inch space around each macaroon).
7. After that, you prepare the chocolate ganache while the macaroons are setting.
8. Then in a small pan on medium heat, mix together the coconut milk, maple syrup, and carob powder.
9. Drizzle a small amount of chocolate ganache over each macaroon.
10. Finally, you place the tray of chocolate covered macaroons in the fridge for 30 minutes.
11. You can serve chilled with a nice cup of tea.

Serves: 4

Ingredients

½ cup of cold leaf lard (snow white, odorless lard best for pastries)

1 tablespoon of maple syrup

1 cup of cassava flour

4 tablespoons of ice cold water

Directions:

1. Meanwhile, you heat oven to 450 degrees F.
2. After which you place flour and lard in food processor.
3. After that, you pulse until crumbs form.
4. Then you add water and maple syrup, pulse until a ball forms.
5. At this point, you place four small tart pans on a baking sheet.
6. This is when you divide dough into four balls.
7. Furthermore, you use fingers or a tart tamper to mold dough into tart pans.
8. After that, you prick dough all over with fork.
9. Finally, you bake for 12 minutes.
10. Then you remove and allow cooling completely.

Sweet Potato Filling

Serves: 4

Ingredients

⅓ Cup of full-fat coconut milk

½ teaspoons of cinnamon

¼ teaspoon of mace

1 teaspoon of tapioca

⅛ Cup of boiling water

1 cup of sweet potato (chopped)

¼ cup of maple syrup

½ teaspoon of ginger

¼ teaspoon of sea salt

½ tablespoon of gelatin

Directions:

1. First, while tart shells are baking, peel and chop one small sweet potato.
2. After which you boil until fork tender, about 10 minutes; drain.
3. After that, you place all ingredients, except gelatin and water, in food processor.
4. You process on high for about 30 seconds.
5. At this point, you place gelatin in a shallow dish, pour boiling water over and stir until gelatin is completely dissolved.
6. This is when you pour gelatin into filling mixture and process on high for 30 more seconds.
7. Finally, you pour filling into cooled tart shells. Place into refrigerator to set.

Serves: 4

Ingredients

¾ cup of full-fat coconut milk

1 teaspoon of alcohol-free vanilla

¼ cup of honey

1 tablespoon of palm shortening

Directions:

1. First, while filling is setting, combine all ingredients in small sauce pan.
2. After which you bring to a rapid boil, stirring occasionally.
3. After that, you let boil for about 20 minutes or until mixture has the consistency of caramel sauce and then allow cooling in refrigerator for 10 minutes.
4. Then you take tarts out, drizzle with caramel, and sprinkle with sea salt.

Notes

Remember that this recipe makes about 4 tarts, but half a tart is easily a serving for 1 individual, resulting in 8 servings.

Strawberry-Orange Sorbet
Serves: 8-12 servings

Ingredients

2 cups of orange juice

¼ cup of honey (it is optional)

4 cups of strawberries (sliced)

Directions:

1. First, you combine all ingredients in a blender and process until smooth.
2. Then you run through an ice cream maker according to the manufacturer's instructions.

Strawberry Balsamic Ice Cream

Serves: 4-8 servings

Ingredients

½ cup of maple syrup (divided)

3 tablespoons of balsamic vinegar

One (13.5-ounce) can coconut milk

1 pint strawberries (hulled and sliced)

½ cup of basil (packed)

1 teaspoon of vanilla extract

Directions:

1. Meanwhile, you heat the oven to 375 degrees F.
2. After which you combine the strawberries, ¼ cup maple syrup, balsamic vinegar, and vanilla in a bowl and toss to combine.
3. After that, you line a baking dish or jelly roll sheet with parchment paper or a silicone liner.
4. Then you pour the strawberries into a single layer in the dish.
5. At this point, you bake 30 minutes, stirring once halfway through, then let cool to room temperature.
6. This is when you puree the strawberries with the coconut milk, remaining maple syrup, and basil in a blender until smooth.
7. Furthermore, you chill at least 30 minutes, then run through your ice cream maker according to the manufacturer's instructions.
8. Remember, if you don't have an ice cream maker but do have a high-powered blender, after pureeing the ingredients the first time, transfer to the freezer for 30 minutes, then puree again.
9. Finally, you freeze another 30 minutes and puree one more time, then freeze.

Thyme-Scented Strawberry Fool

Serves: 6 servings

Ingredients

3 tablespoons of honey (divided)

1½ lbs. of strawberries, hulled and quartered, halved if already small

3 large thyme sprigs

Cream from the top of two 400-ml cans coconut milk (NOTE: will yield 1½-2 cups)

Directions:

1. First, you place the strawberries, thyme and 1 tablespoon of honey into a large pan.
2. After which you cook on a medium heat until juices begin to emerge, then you turn the heat down to low and continue cooking, uncovered, until softened and an almost syrupy jam-like consistency, about 12-15 minutes.
3. After that, you taste a bit of the syrup to see how thyme-y the flavor is and either leaves it in for a more pronounced flavor as it cools or discards it, depending on your preference.
4. At this point, you pour the mixture into a bowl and set aside to cool completely.
5. This is when you turn the cans of refrigerated coconut milk upside down, open with a can opener and slowly pour the watery liquid off into a separate jug (NOTE: you can use this liquid for smoothies or drink as is).
6. Furthermore, you scoop out the cream that is left below, which should be between 1½ and 2 cups, and put into a mixing bowl.
7. Then using a stand mixer or a hand held, whip the cream and remaining 2 tablespoons of honey into soft, pillow peaks.
8. In addition, you discard the thyme sprigs if you left them in and fold in the strawberries and syrup, reserving a small amount for garnishing.
9. After that, you spoon into glasses or pretty dishes and put into the refrigerator until you are ready to serve.
10. Finally, you decorate with the reserved strawberries immediately before serving.
11. This recipe will still be okay to eat the next day if kept in the refrigerator.

Notes

Remember to put 2 cans of coconut milk in the fridge at least the night before you want to make the fool.

Lemon-Raspberry Gelatin Gummies

Serves: 24 gummies

Ingredients

1 cup of frozen raspberries

¼ cup of grass-fed gelatin

¾ cup of lemon juice

3 tablespoons of honey

Directions:

1. First, you place lemon juice and raspberries in a blender and blend on high until completely mixed.
2. After which you pour into a saucepan.
3. After that, you add the honey and gelatin and whisk together (NOTE: You will have a thick paste).
4. Then you turn the heat on low, and continue to whisk the mixture for about 5-10 minutes, until it becomes thin and everything is incorporated.
5. This is when you take off the heat.
6. Furthermore, you pour into silicone molds or a small baking dish.
7. Finally, you set in the refrigerator for at least 1 hour to firm up.
8. Remember that if you use a small baking dish as a receptacle, cut into bite-size squares. Otherwise, remove gummies from their molds and enjoy!

Gingersnap Cookies

Serves: 12-14 cookies

Ingredients

1½ cups of arrowroot starch/flour

½ tablespoon of maple syrup

1½ teaspoons of grated fresh ginger

⅛ Teaspoon of ground cloves

¼ cup of coconut sugar (it is optional)

2 cups of pitted dates (soaked in hot water for five minutes and then drained)

¼ cup of blackstrap molasses

2 tablespoons of coconut oil or lard

1 teaspoon of cinnamon

⅛ Teaspoon of sea salt

Directions:

1. Meanwhile, you heat the oven to 325 degrees.
2. After which you place the strained dates, arrowroot, maple syrup, molasses, coconut oil or lard, spices, and sea salt in a food processor.
3. After that, you process just until everything is just incorporated - you will still have little flecks of date and ginger (NOTE: I like to use the pulse function on my processor to make sure it doesn't get over mixed).
4. At this point, you place the coconut sugar (it is optional) on a small plate.
5. This is when you take a tablespoon and a half of dough, form it into a ball, and smash one side of it into the sugar, forming a 2-inch, flat cookie.
6. Then you place on a cookie sheet lined with parchment paper.
7. Furthermore, you bake for about 20-25 minutes, until they darken in color and are slightly more browned on the bottom.
8. Finally, you transfer to a cooling rack and let cool for 10 minutes before enjoying.

Notes

Storage: make sure you keep sealed in an airtight container for a week at room temperature.

Summer Blackberry Pie

Serves: 6-8

Ingredients

Ingredients for the Crust:

1 cup of arrowroot flour

½ cup of cold water

1 cup of coconut flour

¼ teaspoon of sea salt

¾ cup of coconut oil

Ingredients for the Filling:

6 cups of fresh blackberries (rinsed and drained)

½ lemons (juiced)

¼ cup honey

Directions:

Meanwhile, you heat your oven to 325 degrees.

Directions on how to make the crust:

1. First, you combine the coconut flour, arrowroot flour, and sea salt in a large bowl.
2. After which you cut in the coconut oil with a pastry cutter or stand mixer until you have pea-sized granules.
3. After that, you add the cold water, little by little, and mix until the dough is just moist enough to all stick together (**NOTE:** it will still be pretty crumbly, not like regular dough).
4. At this point, you place in a 9-inch deep pie dish, and spread evenly across the bottoms and sides using your fingers.
5. Then you prick some holes around the bottom with a fork, and bake for 20 minutes, or until lightly browned.
6. Furthermore, while the crust is baking, I suggest you place 3 cups of the blackberries and the lemon juice in a small saucepan on medium heat.
7. After which you bring to a boil and then turn to low.
8. Then you cook for about 20-30 minutes, or until the mixture has reduced and thickened.
9. In addition, you take off the heat, stir in the honey and add the remaining blackberries.

10. This is when you pour into the baked pie crust, spreading it evenly into the corners.
11. After that, you turn up the heat to 350, and bake for another 10 minutes.
12. Finally, you remove from the oven and let cool before serving.

Coconut-Raspberry "Cheesecake"

NOTE: The cake must be allowed to set in the refrigerator for at least 12 hours. Originally posted

Serves: 12

Ingredients

Ingredients for the Crust:

3 cups of dates (pitted and soaked for 5 minutes in warm water)

1 cup of coconut oil (melted)

⅓ Cup of coconut flour

⅓ Cup of unsweetened coconut flakes ⅛ teaspoon salt

Ingredients for the Filling:

1½ cups of coconut concentrate

5 cups of frozen raspberries

1½ teaspoons of vanilla extract

Thick coconut flakes (for garnish)

1½ cups of raw honey

1 cup of coconut oil

6 tablespoons of tapioca starch

¼ teaspoon of salt

Fresh raspberries (for garnish)

Directions:

First, you place the jars of coconut oil, coconut concentrate and raw honey in a pan with very hot water in order to let them soften.

How to prepare the crust:

1. Meanwhile, you heat your oven to 325 degrees.
2. After which you strain the dates and place in a food processor or high-powered blender with the melted coconut oil.
3. After that, you blend for 30 seconds or so until a chunky paste forms.

NOTE: Be warned you may have to stop and scrape the sides if you are using a blender, and the oil will not completely mix with the dates, but the crust will still turn out fine.

4. At this point, you combine the coconut flour, shredded coconut and salt in a bowl.
5. This is when you add the date paste and mix thoroughly.
6. Furthermore, you place the mixture into the bottom of an 8" spring-form pan, pressing the mixture down evenly.
7. Then you use a small spatula to clean up the top edge around the sides of the pan, where the filling will meet the crust.
8. In addition, you bake for 30-35 minutes, until the crust browns and hardens a little bit (NOTE: The texture will still be soft until it finishes cooling).
9. Finally, you set aside while you make the filling.

How to make the filling:

1. First, you combine the raw honey, coconut concentrate, coconut oil, and frozen raspberries in a saucepan on low heat.
2. After which you stir until the raspberries are no longer frozen and the mixture is warm, about 5 minutes.
3. After that, you transfer to a blender and add the tapioca starch, vanilla extract, and salt.
4. Then you blend on high for about a minute, until completely mixed.
5. At this point, you pour carefully into the spring-form pan on top of the crust.
6. This is when you set in the refrigerator undisturbed for at least 12 hours to allow the cake to cool and completely harden.
7. Finally, when it is solid, carefully remove the spring-form pan.
8. Then you decorate the top of the cake with thick flake coconut chips and fresh raspberries.

Pineapple-Lime Popsicles

Serves: 8-10

Ingredients

1/4 cup of lime juice

Pinch of sea salt

3 cups of ripe pineapple (roughly chopped)

You will also need:

Popsicle molds

food-grade Popsicle stick

High-powered blender

Directions:

1. First, you combine the pineapple, lime juice and sea salt in a blender and blend on high for a minute, to thoroughly mix.
2. After which you fill your Popsicle molds with the mixture, making sure to leave a little space at the top of each one to give them some room to expand as they freeze.

NOTE: I prefer to let them freeze for about 20-30 minutes before putting the Popsicle sticks in so that they don't fall all of the way in as they set.

I suggest you give those 6 hours or so in the freezer.

It will make about 8-10 popsicles.

Note: however, the pulp always seems to separate from the pineapple and lime juice when I make these, but I still think they taste great and love keeping it. If you want, I will suggest you substitute 2½ cups of pineapple juice for the fresh pineapple and they will be more uniform.

Cucumber and Dill Summer Soup
Serves: 4-8

Ingredients

1 avocado (pitted and peeled)

½ cup of filtered water

1 tablespoon of fresh (chopped basil)

½ teaspoon of sea salt

2 cucumbers (peeled and chopped)

1 cup of full-fat coconut milk

3 tablespoons of fresh (chopped dill)

1 teaspoon of grated lemon zest

Juice from 1 lemon

Make sure you reserve some cucumber, avocado, dill, and lemon if you would like to fix appetizers as pictured

Directions:

1. First, you puree all ingredients in blender or food processor until smooth.
2. Then for an extra smooth soup, I suggest you pour through fine mesh sieve to filter out extra vegetable fibers.
3. Finally, you chill and serve with shredded chicken or shrimp as main dish or garnished as appetizer.

Sweet Potato and Lime Soup with Coconut and Chives

Serves: 4

Ingredients

1 large onion (thinly sliced)

2 plump cloves garlic (minced)

3 cups of chicken bone broth

Juice of 2 large limes (6 tablespoons)

Swirl of coconut milk (it is optional)

1 tablespoon of fat (coconut oil)

2 stalks celery (chopped)

2½ lb. of orange sweet potatoes (peeled and roughly chopped)

Zest of 1 large lime

1 teaspoon Maldon sea salt

Snipped chives

Directions:

1. First, you heat fat in a large saucepan and add onion.
2. After which you sweat it gently for about 6-8 minutes until softened and translucent, then add the celery and garlic and cook for a further 2-3 minutes.
3. After that, you add sweet potatoes to the pan, together with bone broth and lime zest and bring to a simmer.
4. Then you cover and cook for about 15-18 minutes until sweet potatoes are tender.
5. At this point, you remove from heat and stir in lime juice.
6. Furthermore, working in batches, you transfer soup to a blender and blend until completely smooth, making sure to leave the feeder cap open so that steam can escape and your walls remain the color they are supposed to be!
7. After that, you return soup to the pan and reheat if necessary.
8. This is when you taste and add salt, adjusting the quantity to suit your own palate.
9. Finally, you pour into warmed bowls, swirl a little coconut milk on the top if you like, scatter over some snipped chives and serve.

Zesty Green "Sick" Soup

Serves: 4

Ingredients

1 large onion (chopped)

2-in piece ginger (peeled and minced)

1 medium white sweet potato, cubed (about 3 cups)

1 bunch kale (chopped)

½ teaspoon of sea salt

1 bunch of cilantro

2 tablespoons of solid cooking fat (coconut oil works great here)

3 cloves garlic (minced)

3 cups of bone broth

2 small/ one large head of broccoli, chopped (about 1 cup)

One lemon, ½ zested and juice reserved

Avocado for garnish

Directions:

1. First, you place the fat in the bottom of a heavy-bottomed pot on medium heat.
2. Then when the fat has melted and the pan is hot, add the onions, and cook, stirring, for 5-7 minutes, or until lightly browned and translucent.
3. After which you add the garlic and ginger, and cook for another minute, or until fragrant.
4. After that, you add the bone broth, sweet potato, and broccoli to the pot and bring to a boil.
5. At this point, you turn down to a simmer, cover, and cook for about 10-15 minutes, or until the vegetables are tender.
6. Furthermore, you turn off the heat; add the kale, half of the bunch of cilantro, lemon zest and juice, and sea salt.
7. After which you let cool for a few minutes, and blend with a high-powered blender or immersion blender until smooth.
8. Finally, you serve warm garnished with avocado and cilantro.

Note: make sure you keep for a week in the refrigerator and freezes well.

Orange-Tarragon Beet Soup
Serves: 2-4

Ingredients

Filtered water to cover

1 tablespoon of grated orange peel (however, any orange variety is fine, I used mandarins)

1 tablespoon of red wine vinegar

½ cup of full-fat coconut milk

3 large or better still 4-6 small beets (peeled and diced)

1 tablespoon of minced, fresh tarragon

1 tablespoon of olive oil

1 teaspoon of sea salt

Directions:

1. First, you place beets in pot, cover with water, bring to a boil.
2. After which you reduce to simmer, add tarragon and orange peel.
3. After that, you simmer until beets are fork tender, about 30 minutes.
4. At this point, you add oil, vinegar, sea salt, and coconut milk to high-powered blender or food processor
5. Then when beets are done, add them without draining to blender or food processor (be sure your appliance is heat-proof).
6. Finally, you process on high until completely smooth. Serve and enjoy!
7. Remember that this recipe makes 2 main dish servings or 4 side servings.

Cream of Avocado Soup with Crab Meat

Serves: 3 cups

Ingredients

2 tablespoons of chopped shallots or better still red onions

2 tablespoons of full fat coconut cream (from a refrigerated can of coconut milk)

¼ teaspoon of sea salt (or more to taste)

1 tablespoon of chopped chives for garnish

3 ripe avocados

1½ tablespoons of lemon juice

1½ cups of chicken broth or bone broth

1 can crab meat (about 6 oz. /170 g), drained

Directions:

1. First, you put the avocado pulp, shallots, lemon juice, coconut cream, chicken broth, and sea salt in a high speed blender.
2. After which you mix on high for 30 seconds, until the mixture becomes smooth and creamy.
3. After that, you chill for at least 1 hour in the refrigerator.
4. Then you serve the cream of avocado chilled with a portion of crab meat on top and some chives for the garnish.

Summer Fruit Gazpacho

Serves: 6

Ingredients

Ingredients For the gazpacho:

2 lbs. of strawberries

½ medium watermelons (approx. 10 inches across)

Ingredients For the raspberry sauce:

1 tablespoon of lemon juice

4 tablespoon of full fat coconut milk (from a can)

6 oz. of raspberries

Zest of 1 organic lemon

Mint leaves and some coconut milk (for garnish)

Directions:

1. First, you scoop out all the pulp from the watermelon with a spoon and place in a large pot.
2. After which you keep the skin of the watermelon and save in the refrigerator for later.
3. After that, you stem and quarter the strawberries.
4. At this point, you add to the watermelon.
5. Then with a hand-held mixer, mix the watermelon and strawberries until you obtain a smooth cream; set aside.
6. This is when you mash the raspberries with a fork in a small bowl.
7. Finally, you add the lemon juice, lemon zest, and coconut milk. Mix well.

Directions on how to serve:

1. However, this gazpacho is best served chilled.
2. If you prepare in advance, I suggest you keep the soup and raspberry sauce in the refrigerator until it is time to serve.
3. Remember that for a pretty presentation, you may serve the gazpacho in the skin of the watermelon! For each person, I suggest you pour 2 ladles of gazpacho in a soup dish, drop a portion of raspberry sauce in the middle, and decorate with a few mint leaves and a drizzle of coconut milk.

Zuppa Toscana
Serves: 4-6 servings

Ingredients

1 small onion (chopped)

2 cloves garlic (minced)

1 large celeriac (peeled and chopped)

⅓ Cup of coconut milk

6 slices bacon

1 lb. of ground beef

4 cups of bone broth

2 cups of kale (chopped)

Directions:

1. First, you cook the bacon in a stock pot over medium heat until crispy.
2. After which you remove it from the pan, leaving the bacon fat behind.
3. After that, you add the onion and cook for about 3 minutes until translucent.
4. Add the ground beef and cook, stirring, for about 3 minutes until browned.
5. At this point, you add the garlic and cook, stirring, another 2-3 minutes.
6. This is when you add the broth and celeriac and bring to a boil.
7. Furthermore, you reduce the heat to a simmer and cook, uncovered, 20 minutes or until the celeriac is tender.
8. Then you add the kale and coconut milk and cook until the kale wilts.
9. Finally, you serve topped with crumbled bacon.

Dandelion Pesto
Serves: 1½ cups

Ingredients

½ cup of olive oil (with an extra ¼ cup optional)

½ lemons (juiced)

1 large bunch of dandelion greens

3 cloves garlic (peeled)

½ teaspoon of sea salt

Directions:

1. First, you wash the dandelion greens in a colander, removing any leaves or stems that are expired or wilted.
2. After which you place in a food processor with the olive oil, garlic, sea salt and lemon.
3. After that, you process until desired consistency is reached, adding additional olive oil if the mixture is too thick.
4. Finally, you use stirred into soups, eaten on plantain crackers, or mixed with stir-fried vegetables.

Notes

Make sure you keep in the refrigerator for about a week.

Serves: 6

Ingredients

2 tablespoons of solid cooking fat (coconut oil, duck fat, lard, or tallow)

4 cloves garlic (minced)

1½ teaspoons of sea salt

1½ cups of coconut milk

Dandelion pesto (to taste)

2 acorn squash (with ends trimmed, halved, and de-seeded)

1 yellow onion (chopped)

1-inch piece ginger (peeled and minced)

1½ cups of bone broth

Directions:

1. Meanwhile, you heat the oven to 400 degrees.
2. After which you place the acorn squash face up on a baking sheet and cook for 40 minutes, or until a fork can pierce through the flesh easily.
3. After that, you let cool for 20 minutes, and then peel the skin off with your hands.
4. Then you roughly chop and set aside to add to the soup later.
5. At this point, you heat the solid cooking fat in the bottom of a heavy-bottomed pot.
6. Then when the fat has melted and the pan is hot, add the onions and cook, stirring, for 8 minutes, or until they are lightly browned and translucent.
7. This is when you add the garlic, ginger and sea salt and cook, stirring, for a minute or two, until fragrant.
8. Furthermore, you add the bone broth and squash to the pot and bring to a boil and then turn down to a simmer and cook for about 10 minutes, until the squash starts to break up.
9. After that, you turn off the heat and carefully blend the soup in batches, returning to the pot when finished.
10. Then you stir in the coconut milk.
11. Finally, you serve garnished with a tablespoon or two of dandelion pesto.

Notes

Make sure you keep in the refrigerator for about a week. Also freezes well!

Magic "Chili"
Serves: 6

Ingredients

1 large onion (chopped)

4 cups of bone broth

3 carrots, chopped into 1½-inch pieces (about 2 cups)

2 tablespoons of fresh oregano (minced)

½ teaspoon of sea salt

⅛ Teaspoon of cinnamon

1 tablespoon of solid cooking fat (coconut oil, lard, tallow, duck fat)

4 cloves garlic (minced)

2 parsnips, chopped into 1½-inch pieces (about 2 cups)

1 large beet, grated (about 2 cups)

1 teaspoon of onion powder

½ teaspoon of garlic powder

2 pounds of grass-fed ground beef

A few parsley sprigs, for garnish

Directions:

1. First, you heat the solid cooking fat in a heavy-bottomed pot on medium-high heat.
2. When the fat has melted and the pan is hot, I suggest you add the onions, and cook, stirring for 7 minutes, or until the onions are translucent.
3. After which you add the garlic and cook for another 3 minutes.
4. After that, you add the bone broth, carrots, parsnips, grated beet, and all of the spices except for the parsley.
5. Then you bring to a boil; turn down to a simmer, and cook, covered, for 20 minutes.
6. In the meantime, brown the ground beef in a skillet over medium high heat, being sure to stir it occasionally so that it is browned evenly.
7. In addition, you add the ground beef to the vegetables and simmer, covered, for another 15 minutes.
8. Finally, you serve garnished with fresh parsley.

Cream of Broccoli Soup

Serves: 4

Ingredients

One large yellow onion

One large rutabaga (about ¾ pound), cut into 1-inch chunks

1 lb. of broccoli, florets and stems (chopped)

1 cup of water

1 avocado (for garnish)

1 tablespoon of solid cooking fat

4 cloves garlic (minced)

3 cups of bone broth

1 cup of mushrooms (thinly sliced)

1 teaspoon of sea salt

1½ cups of coconut milk (about 1 can)

Directions:

1. First, you heat the solid cooking fat in the bottom of a heavy-bottomed pot.
2. When the fat is melted and the pan is hot, I suggest you add the onion and cook for 8 minutes, stirring, until translucent.
3. After which you add the garlic and continue to cook, stirring for another couple of minutes.
4. After that, you add the rutabaga and bone broth, bring to a boil, and turn down to a simmer.
5. At this point, you cook, covered for 10 minutes.
6. Then you add the broccoli, mushrooms, water, and salt to the pot and bring back to a boil.
7. Furthermore, you turn down to a simmer, and cook, covered for another 10-15 minutes - until all of the vegetables are just soft.
8. After that, you add the coconut milk to the pot and stir to combine.
9. This is when you turn off the heat and carefully transfer some of the soup to a blender.

(**NOTE:** for me I prefer to transfer more rutabaga chunks and broccoli stems and leave the florets in the soup).

10. At this point, you blend for a few seconds until well incorporated.
11. Then you add back to the soup, blending another batch if you would like it less chunky (for me I prefer to leave some chunks instead of blending the whole thing, but it is up to you!).
12. Finally, you garnish with fresh avocado and serve.

Storage: make sure you keep well in the refrigerator for a few days, without the avocado. Also freezes well.

Serves: 4

Ingredients

1 large fennel bulb (ends removed and sliced thinly)

1-inch piece ginger (peeled and minced)

3 cups of bone broth

2 tablespoons of coconut oil

2 cloves garlic (minced)

2 pounds beets (peeled and cut into 1½-inch chunks)

1 bay leaf

½ teaspoon of salt

Fennel fronds (for garnish)

Directions:

1. First, you heat the coconut oil and sauté the fennel in a heavy-bottomed pot for about 12 minutes, or until it softens.
2. After which you add the ginger and garlic to the pot and cook for a few more minutes, stirring.
3. After that, you add the broth, beets, bay leaf, and salt.
4. Then you bring to a boil, cover, and turn down to a simmer.
5. At this point, you cook for 1 hour 15 minutes, or until the beets are tender.
6. Furthermore, in a high-powered blender or food processor, blend until desired consistency is reached, adding more broth if needed.
7. Finally, you serve warm, with fennel fronds to garnish.

AIP Carrot and Sweet Potato "Chili"
Serves: 5-6

Ingredients

1 onion (chopped)

1 tablespoon of fresh thyme

4 cups of sweet potatoes (cut into large chunks)

1 teaspoon of sea salt

Cilantro for garnish

2 tablespoons of solid cooking fat

8 cloves of garlic (minced)

2 cups of carrots (cut into large chunks)

4 cups of bone broth

2 pounds of grass-fed ground beef

1-2 avocados

Directions:

1. First, you heat your cooking fat in the bottom of a heavy-bottomed pot.
2. After which you add the onion and cook for a few minutes, until translucent.
3. After that, you add the garlic and thyme and cook for another couple of minutes, stirring.
4. At this point, you add the carrots and sweet potatoes and cook for 5 minutes, or until gently browned.
5. This is when you add the bone broth and sea salt and bring to a boil, cover and then simmer for 20 minutes, until the vegetables are soft.
6. In the meantime, cook the ground beef in a skillet until thoroughly cooked throughout and browned; set aside.
7. Then when the vegetables are finished, add the ground beef and stir to combine.
8. In addition, you continue cooking for another 15 minutes covered at a simmer.
9. Finally, you serve each bowl garnished with avocado slices and fresh parsley.

Parsnip and Pear Soup with Fried Sage

Ingredients

1 large yellow onion (chopped)

2 cloves garlic (minced)

2 pounds parsnips (chopped into 1½-inch chunks)

¼ cup of fresh sage (chopped)

3 tablespoons of solid cooking fat

2-inch piece ginger (peeled and minced)

4 cups of bone broth

1 large, firm pear, cored and chopped into 1½-inch chunks

½ teaspoon of sea salt

Directions:

1. First, you heat 1 tablespoon of the solid cooking fat in a heavy-bottomed pot over medium heat.
2. Then when the pot is warm and the fat has melted, add the onion and cook, stirring occasionally, for 8 minutes.
3. After which you add the garlic and ginger, and cook, stirring, for another couple of minutes, or until fragrant.
4. After that, you add the bone broth and parsnips bring to a boil, turn down to a simmer, and let cook, covered, for 10 minutes.
5. Furthermore, add the pear and salt and let cook for another 5-10 minutes, until the parsnips and pear are just soft.
6. In the meantime, heat the rest of the solid cooking fat in a small skillet on medium-high heat.
7. Then when the pan is hot and the fat has melted, you add the fresh sage and fry for about 5-10 minutes, stirring and flipping the sage.

NOTE: the sage is finished cooking when it no longer bubbles and has absorbed most of the oil in the pan; they should be fairly crispy.

8. Finally, you blend the soup on high to create a thick puree, add salt to taste if needed, and serve garnished with fried sage.

Storage: make sure you keep in the refrigerator for about a week. It freezes well.

Chicken Soup with Acorn Squash

Serves: 6

Ingredients

1 onion (chopped)

2 cloves of garlic

4 large carrots (chopped)

1 large or better still 2 small acorn squash (peeled, seeded and cut into 1-1/2 inch cubes)

1 (4-5 pound) stewing hen or better still rooster

1 bay leaf

1 tablespoon of salt

4 stalks celery (chopped)

1 tablespoon of coconut oil

Added salt to taste

Directions:

1. First, begin by cleaning the chicken and placing it in a large stock pot.
2. After which you add the onion, bay leaf, garlic, salt and half of the carrots and celery.
3. After that, you fill the pot with water until the chicken is just covered.
4. At this point, you bring to a boil and then lower to a simmer, and cook until the meat is tender, about 1-2 hours depending on the size of your bird.
5. This is when you skim the surface of the broth to remove any scum that may appear during cooking.
6. Then you remove the chicken and skim the broth, discarding the vegetables.
7. Furthermore, in the empty stock pot, bring the coconut oil to medium-heat and add the remaining vegetables (acorn squash, carrots, and celery).
8. After which you cook until browned on the edges (about 10 minutes).
9. Then you add the broth back to the pot, and simmer for 20 minutes.
10. In addition, while the vegetables are simmering, remove the meat from the chicken carcass and place into a bowl.
11. Finally, you add the chicken back to the soup and simmer another 20-30 minutes, or until the vegetables are tender.
12. After which you add more salt to taste.

"Sick Soup"
Serves: 4 quarts

Ingredients

1 quart filtered water

1 pound of green beans (roughly chopped)

1 bunch of leafy greens (like kale or chard), roughly chopped

2-inch piece of ginger (peeled and chopped)

Salt (to taste)

Coconut oil (to taste)

2 quarts of bone broth

3 sweet potatoes (sub squash for low-fodmaps), cut into chunks

2 zucchini (roughly chopped)

4 cloves garlic (peeled and chopped)

1 avocado (sliced thinly)

Lemon juice (to taste)

Directions:

1. First, you place the bone broth and water in a large stock pot on medium-high.
2. Then when it comes to a boil, turn down to a simmer and adds the sweet potatoes or squash and cook for 20-30 minutes or until tender.
3. After which you turn the heat off and add the green beans, zucchini and leafy green vegetables to the still-hot water.
4. After that, you cover and let the soup sit for a few minutes.
5. At this point, you salt the soup to taste and add the garlic and ginger.
6. Finally, you blend the soup in batches and place in another pot.

NOTE: for me I like to serve with a avocado slices, a scoop of coconut oil, a squeeze of lemon and some more salt on top.

Celeriac Leek Soup
Serves: 4

Ingredients

2 leeks (ends removed and sliced thinly)

1-inch piece ginger (minced)

2 pounds of celeriac (peeled and cut into 1 ½ inch chunks)

½ teaspoon of salt

4 slices of sugar-free, pastured bacon

3 cloves garlic (minced)

4 cups of bone broth

1 tablespoon of apple-cider vinegar

A few sprigs of parsley

Directions:

1. First, you heat a heavy-bottomed pot on medium heat; when it is ready, cook the bacon until crispy, turning a couple times.
2. After which you remove the bacon to cool and leave the fat in the bottom of the pan.
3. After that, you add the leeks and cook for a few minutes, stirring.
4. Then you add the garlic and ginger and cook for another couple of minutes.
5. At this point, you add the broth, celeriac, apple-cider vinegar and salt and bring to a boil.
6. This is when you turn down to a simmer, cover, and cook for 15 minutes, or until celeriac is soft.
7. While the soup is cooking, I will suggest you crumble the bacon.
8. Furthermore, you transfer to a blender and process until desired consistency is reached, adding more bone broth if needed.
9. Finally, you serve with parsley and crumbled bacon on top.

Beef and Butternut Stew with Pear and Thyme
Serves: 4-6

Ingredients

2-3 pound roast or better still stew meat (I used sirloin tip) cut into 1½" cubes

5 cloves garlic (minced)

2 cups of bone broth

¼ teaspoon of cinnamon

2 pears (chopped)

1 tablespoon of fresh thyme

1½ tablespoons of coconut oil

1 onion (chopped)

2 inch piece ginger (minced)

1 butternut squash (peeled and cubed)

½ teaspoon of sea salt

1 cup of mushrooms (sliced)

Directions:

1. First, you heat 1 tablespoon of the coconut oil in a heavy-bottomed pot on medium-high heat and brown the meat on all sides.
2. After which you remove from the pot, and turn the heat down to medium.
3. After that, you add the onion and cook for about 5 minutes or until they begin to soften.
4. Then you add the ginger and garlic, and cook for another couple of minutes, being careful to stir them gently so that they don't burn.
5. At this point, you add the bone broth or stock and the browned meat to the pot, and bring to a simmer on low.
6. This is when you cover tightly and cook for 15 minutes, making sure to keep it at a simmer.
7. Furthermore, you add the butternut squash, cinnamon, and sea salt and simmer covered another 15 minutes.
8. This is when you add the pears and simmers for another 30 minutes or until the meat and squash is both tender.

9. In addition, you heat the rest of the coconut oil on high heat in a small skillet and cook the mushrooms for about 5 minutes, or until browned and tender.
10. Finally, when the stew is done, garnish with sautéed mushrooms and fresh thyme.

Simple Asian-Inspired Stir-Fry

Serves: 4 servings

Ingredients

1 lb. of chicken or beef, sliced (it is optional)

¼ cup of apple cider vinegar

6 tablespoons of coconut aminos

½ teaspoon of garlic powder

2 lbs. of stir-fry vegetables (chopped)

1 cup of broth

⅛ Cup of honey

½ teaspoon of sea salt

¾ teaspoon of ground ginger

Directions:

1. First, you combine all ingredients in a large stock pot over high heat and bring to a boil.
2. After which you reduce the heat to medium, cover the pot, and simmer for 20 minutes or until the vegetables are fork-tender and the meat is cooked through.
3. Then you serve hot.

Serves: 8-12 servings

Ingredients

1 teaspoon of sea salt

1 teaspoon of ground ginger

½ cup of your favorite AIP-friendly "tomato" sauce or better still BBQ sauce

½ yellow squash (sliced)

3 ounces of olives (sliced)

3 pounds of ground meat

1 teaspoon of dried oregano

1 dash ground cinnamon

½ zucchini (sliced)

4 ounces mushrooms (sliced)

Directions:

1. Meanwhile, you heat the oven to 350 degrees F.
2. After which you combine the ground meat and spices and mix well.
3. After that, you line a rimmed baking sheet with parchment paper or a silicone liner.
4. Then you spread the meat over the sheet, flattening it evenly to about ¼ inch.
5. At this point, you bake for 10 minutes or until cooked through.
6. This is when you transfer to a pizza stone or a wire rack on top of a baking sheet.
7. Finally, you add the sauce and toppings, then return to the oven for 10 minutes or until the toppings are cooked.

Rosemary and Garlic Beef Liver Appetizer

Serves: 8

Ingredients

8 oz. (about 226 gr) beef liver, cut into 8 pieces

2 teaspoons of fresh rosemary (chopped)

1½ cups of arugula

2 tablespoons of olive oil

Salt to taste

2 teaspoons of fresh garlic (crushed and minced)

2 apples

Direction:

1. First, in a large skillet, warm the olive oil on medium heat.
2. After which you add liver, salt, garlic, and rosemary.
3. After that, you cover and cook for 5 minutes, turning the liver over to brown on both sides.
4. At this point, you remove from the heat and set aside to rest for 5 minutes.
5. In the meantime, you cut the apples crosswise to obtain 8 round slices of ¼-inch thick.
6. On a serving platter, you place the apples, some arugula and pieces of liver on top.
7. Then you garnish with a little bit of olive oil, rosemary, and garlic spooned out of the skillet.

Citrus Braised Lamb Shoulder
Serves: 4

Ingredients

2-3 lb. of lamb shoulder roast, bone-in

1 onion (diced)

1 orange (zest reserved and juiced)

1½ lbs. of carrots (cut into 1½-inch chunks)

2 tablespoons of solid cooking fat

½ teaspoon of sea salt

2 cups of bone broth

4 sprigs of rosemary

Additional sea salt (to taste)

Directions:

1. Meanwhile, you heat your oven to 325 degrees F.
2. After which you rub the salt all over the outside of the lamb roast.
3. After that, you place the solid cooking fat in the bottom of a heavy-bottomed pot that is oven-safe on medium-high heat.
4. Then when the fat is melted and the pan is hot, add the roast, and brown for about 3-4 minutes a side.
5. At this point, you remove from the pot, turn down the heat, and add the onions.
6. This is when you cook for 5-7 minutes, stirring, until just browned.
7. Furthermore, you add the bone broth, orange juice; rosemary and lamb roast back to the pot, fatty side up.
8. After that, you sprinkle with orange zest, cover, and place in the oven.
9. Then you cook for 1½ hours; remove from the oven and add the carrots, making sure to coat them in the braising liquid.
10. Finally, you place back in the oven to cook for another hour.

NOTE:

1. The roast is finished when it is easily torn apart with a fork, and the vegetables are tender.
2. If you would like, I suggest you remove the lamb and vegetables and reduce the liquid for 10 minutes or so to create a flavorful sauce.

3. In the other hand, if you don't have a heavy-bottomed pot, I suggest you brown the roast in a skillet and transfer to a roasting dish covered with foil to cook in the oven.
4. If you use this method, check periodically to make sure there is enough liquid in the bottom of the pan.

Magic "Chili"

Ingredients

1 large onion (chopped)

4 cups of bone broth

3 carrots, chopped into 1½-inch pieces (about 2 cups)

2 tablespoons of fresh oregano (minced)

½ teaspoon of sea salt

2 pounds of grass-fed ground beef

1 tablespoon of solid cooking fat (coconut oil, tallow, lard, duck fat)

4 cloves garlic (minced)

2 parsnips, chopped into 1½-inch pieces (about 2 cups)

1 (about 2 cups) large beet, grated

1 teaspoon of onion powder

½ teaspoon of garlic powder

⅛ Teaspoon of cinnamon

A few parsley sprigs (for garnish)

Directions:

1. First, you heat the solid cooking fat in a heavy-bottomed pot on medium-high heat.
2. Then when the fat has melted and the pan is hot, add the onions, and cook, stirring for 7 minutes, or until the onions are translucent.
3. After which you add the garlic and cook another 3 minutes.
4. After that, you add the bone broth, parsnips, carrots, grated beet, and all of the spices except for the parsley.
5. At this point, you bring to a boil; turn down to a simmer, and cook, covered, for 20 minutes.
6. In the meantime, brown the ground beef in a skillet over medium high heat, being sure to stir it occasionally so that it is browned evenly.
7. Finally, you add the ground beef to the vegetables and simmer, covered, for another 15 minutes.
8. Then you serve garnished with fresh parsley

Citrus-Bison Meatballs

Ingredients

½ yellow onions (minced)

1 teaspoon of grated ginger

1 tablespoon of thyme

¼ cup of coconut aminos

2 tablespoons of solid cooking fat

3 cloves garlic (minced)

2 pounds of ground bison

½ teaspoon of sea salt

One orange, juiced (about ½ cup)

Directions:

1. First, you heat half of the cooking fat in the bottom of a skillet on medium heat.
2. When the fat is melted and the pan is hot, I suggest you add the onion, and cook, stirring, for 8 minutes, or until translucent.
3. After which you add the garlic and ginger and cook, stirring, for a minute, just until fragrant.
4. After that, you remove from heat and place onion mixture into a bowl.
5. Then you set aside to cool for a few minutes.
6. Furthermore, when the onion mixture has cooled, add it to a large bowl with the ground bison, thyme, and salt.
7. After which you gently mix with your hands until everything is well incorporated.
8. Form into 1-1/2" meatballs (let say about 20 totals).
9. At this point, you place the rest of the cooking fat in the bottom of the skillet you used for the onions on medium heat.
10. Then when the fat is melted and the pan is hot, add the meatballs.
11. This is when you brown for three minutes on one side, flip, and add the orange juice and coconut aminos.
12. In addition, you cook, covered, for 10 minutes, or until cooked throughout. Remove from pan and set aside.
13. After that, you leave the remaining juices in the pan and turn up to medium-high heat.
14. Finally, you let the sauce reduce about ½, about 5-10 minutes.
15. Then you serve on a bed of crispy sweet potato noodles and glazed with sauce and fresh thyme.

Crispy Sweet Potato Noodles

Serves: 2

Ingredients

2 tablespoons of solid cooking fat

Vegetable peeler or better still spiralizer

1 large sweet potato (peeled)

¼ teaspoon of sea salt

Directions:

1. First, you use a vegetable peeler; peel the sweet potato into long, flat ribbons. (Alternately, you could spiralizer it with a vegetable spiralizer).
2. After which you heat half of the solid cooking fat in the bottom of a wok or skillet on medium-high heat.
3. Then when the fat has melted and the pan is hot, add half of the sweet potatoes.
4. After that, you let them cook, stirring, for about 10 minutes, being sure not to stir them too often to ensure that they brown on the bottoms.
5. Finally, you add the other half of the solid cooking fat and repeat with the second batch of noodles.

Slow-Roasted Prime Rib

Serves: 4-6

Ingredients

1 (3-rib) prime rib roast, bone-in but separated from the meat, and tied back up (6-7 pounds)

2 teaspoons of sea salt

Directions:

NOTE: 2 hours before cooking, take the prime rib out of the refrigerator to allow to come completely to room temperature.

1. First, you rub all of the exposed surfaces with the sea salt.
2. Then when you are ready to start cooking, preheat the oven to 200 degrees F.
3. After which you place the meat bone side down on a rack in a roasting dish.
4. After that, you cook for about 4-6 hours, or until an internal thermometer reads 125 degrees (for medium-rare; 135 for medium), keeping in mind that the roast will rise in temperature 5 degrees as it cools.
5. Furthermore, you let the roast cool for 30-45 minutes while you increase the oven temperature to 500 degrees.
6. At this point, you place the roast back in the oven for about 7-10 minutes to let the skin get crispy. Remember to watch it carefully, as it can burn easily! Once you take it out of the oven it only needs a few minutes to cool; the meat on the inside has already rested.

Notes

You can brown the outside of the meat for about 7-10 minutes in a skillet once the meat has rested.

Braised Beef Shanks

Serves: 2-3

Ingredients

Sea salt (to taste)

2 tablespoons of fresh thyme plus a few extra sprigs

2 tablespoons of coconut oil

2-4 beef shanks

8 cloves garlic (chopped)

1 cup of bone broth

½ cup of water

Directions:

1. Meanwhile, you heat your oven to 350 degrees.
2. After which you clean the shanks, pat them dry thoroughly and salt both sides to taste.
3. After that, you heat some of the coconut oil in the bottom of a skillet on medium-high heat.
4. At this point, you sear the shanks for a few minutes a side, adding coconut oil if needed.
5. This is when you place seared shanks in a large baking dish.
6. Furthermore, you turn down the heat on the skillet to medium and add the garlic and thyme leaves.
7. After that, you cook for a couple of minutes, until lightly browned and fragrant.
8. Then you add bone broth and water to the skillet and boil to reduce slightly.
9. In addition, you pour the broth mixture over the shanks, and add the remaining thyme sprigs.
10. Finally, you cover tightly with aluminum foil and braise for 2 hours, or until fork-tender.

Pineapple, Mint and Lamb Kebabs

Serves: 4-6

Ingredients

2 cloves of garlic

½ teaspoon of sea salt

Cinnamon (to taste)

1 large pineapple (chopped into 1½" cubes)

½-inch piece ginger

16-24oz lamb shoulder steak (cut into 1½" cubes)

1 bunch of mint leaves

You will also need:

Wooden or better still a metal skewers

Directions:

1. First, you place 1½ cups of the pineapple cubes, garlic, ginger, and sea salt in a blender and blend until incorporated.
2. After which you place in a container or plastic bag with the lamb and marinate for 1 hour, 2 hours maximum.

NOTE: if you have wooden skewers, I suggest you soak them in water before using so that they don't burn on the grill.

3. Furthermore, when the lamb is finished marinating, remove and discard marinade.
4. After that, you thread the lamb, pineapple, and mint on the skewers, alternating one of each.
5. Then you sprinkle skewers with a dusting of cinnamon.
6. Finally, you grill for 10 minutes or until meat is finished, turning and watching to ensure that they don't burn.

Italian-Spiced 50/50 Sausages
Serves: 8-10 patties

Ingredients

1 pound of pastured ground pork

1 tablespoon of minced fresh thyme

½ teaspoon of garlic powder

1 tablespoon of solid cooking fat (lard, coconut oil, tallow, or duck fat)

1 pound of grass-fed ground beef

1 tablespoon of minced fresh oregano

1 tablespoon of minced fresh parsley (it is optional)

½ teaspoon of sea salt

Directions:

1. First, you place the ground beef, pork, herbs, garlic powder and salt in a large bowl and combine well with your hands.
2. Form into about 8-10 patties and place on a plate.
3. After that, you heat the solid cooking fat in the bottom of a cast-iron skillet or frying pan on medium heat.
4. Furthermore, when the fat is melted and the pan is hot, add patties, cook 10 minutes a side, or until thoroughly cooked.

NOTE: you may have to do this in two batches. Alternately, you can bake them at 400 degrees for about 20 minutes or until they are cooked throughout.

Variation: you can switch up the protein in these you can make them 100% beef or pork, or add some lamb into the mix!

Autoimmune Protocol Meatloaf

Serves: 6-8

Ingredients

1 cup of cauliflower, processed into "rice" with a food processor

1 carrot (peeled and grated)

4 cloves garlic (minced)

2 teaspoons of sea salt

2 egg yolks (feel free to omit if on the elimination diet)

3-4 slices of pastured bacon

1 tablespoon of coconut oil

1 zucchini (peeled and grated)

½ onions (minced)

½ cup of parsley (chopped)

2 tablespoons of fresh thyme and/or marjoram

2 lbs. of ground beef, lamb, or better still pork mixture (I used beef and lamb), room temperature

Directions:

1. Meanwhile, you heat your oven to 350 degrees.
2. After which in a skillet, heat the coconut oil and sauté the onion, zucchini, carrot and cauliflower rice for about 5 minutes, adding the garlic at the very end; let cool.
3. After that, in a large bowl mix the egg yolks with the herbs and spices including the fresh parsley.
4. Then you add the meat and vegetables to the bowl.
5. Furthermore, you mix gently with your hands until just incorporated.
6. After that, you transfer the mixture to a 9*5 loaf pan, making sure to spread it evenly into the corners.
7. At this point, you lay the bacon strips across the top, tucking them in to the ends if they are too long.
8. This is when you cook for about 45-50 minutes, or until the internal temperature reaches 155 degrees.
9. After which you remove from oven and carefully pour off liquid, reserving it to cook veggies in later.

10. Finally, you put the loaf back in the oven for 10 minutes under the broiler to crisp up the bacon.
11. Then you let sit for 10 minutes before slicing.

AIP Carrot and Sweet Potato "Chili"
Serves: 5-6

Ingredients

1 onion (chopped)

1 tablespoon of fresh thyme

4 cups of sweet potatoes (cut into large chunks)

1 teaspoon of sea salt

1-2 avocados

2 tablespoons of solid cooking fat

8 cloves garlic (minced)

2 cups of carrots (cut into large chunks)

4 cups of bone broth

2 pounds of grass-fed ground beef

Cilantro for garnish

Directions:

1. First, you heat your cooking fat in the bottom of a heavy-bottomed pot.
2. After which you add the onion and cook for a few minutes, until translucent.
3. After that, you add the garlic and thyme and cook for another couple of minutes, stirring.
4. At this point, you add the carrots and sweet potatoes and cook for 5 minutes, or until gently browned.
5. Then add the bone broth and sea salt and bring to a boil, cover and then simmer for 20 minutes, until the vegetables are soft.
6. In the meantime, you cook the ground beef in a skillet until thoroughly cooked throughout and browned; set aside.
7. Furthermore, when the vegetables are finished, add the ground beef and stir to combine.
8. After which you continue cooking for another 15 minutes covered at a simmer.
9. Finally, you serve each bowl garnished with avocado slices and fresh parsley.

Citrus and Herb Pot-Roast with Carrots and Parsnips

Serves: 6-8

Ingredients

2-3 pound roast

¾ cup of bone broth

1 orange (juiced)

2 parsnips (cut into 2-inch chunks)

1 bay leaf

3 carrots (cut into 2-inch chunks)

2 tablespoons of apple-cider vinegar

1½ teaspoons of sea salt

1 tablespoon of coconut oil

A few sprigs of fresh herbs (I used rosemary, thyme, and sage)

Directions:

1. Meanwhile, you heat your oven to 300 degrees.
2. After which you heat the coconut oil in the bottom of a heavy-bottomed pot (ideally cast-iron) and brown the roast well on all sides.
3. After that, you turn off the heat, remove the roast from the pot and salt it well.
4. Then you add the bone broth, cider vinegar, orange juice and bay leaf to the pot.
5. At this point, you add the roast back and surround it with the carrots and parsnips.
6. In addition, you generously sprinkle fresh herbs all over the roast and the vegetables.
7. Furthermore, making sure you have a lid that fits properly, braise the roast for about 2-3 hours in the oven, checking periodically to make sure there is enough liquid (**NOTE:** you shouldn't have a problem if the lid seals well).
8. Remember that it is finished when the meat is easily pulled apart with a fork.
9. Finally, you serve with some of the juice from the pot poured over top.

Bacon-Beef Liver Pâté with Rosemary and Thyme
Serves: 2 cups

Ingredients

1 small onion (minced)

1 pound grass-fed beef liver

2 tablespoons of fresh thyme (minced)

Slices of fresh carrot or better still cucumber

6 pieces of uncured bacon

4 cloves garlic (minced)

2 tablespoons of fresh rosemary (minced)

½ cup of coconut oil (melted)

½ teaspoon of sea salt

Directions:

1. First, you cook the bacon slices in a cast-iron pot until crispy.
2. After which you set aside to cool, reserving the grease in the pan to cook the liver.
3. After that, you add the onion and cook for 2 minutes on medium-high.
4. At this point, you add the garlic and cook for a minute.
5. This is when you add the liver, sprinkling with the herbs.
6. Then cook for 3-5 minutes per side, until no longer pink in the center.
7. Furthermore, turn off heat, and place contents into a blender or food processor with the coconut oil and sea salt.
8. After which you process until it forms a thick paste, adding more coconut oil if too thick.
9. Then you cut the cooled bacon strips into little bits and mix with the pâté in a small bowl.
10. Finally, you garnish with some fresh herbs and serve on carrot or cucumber slices.

Cranberry-Braised Short Ribs

Serves: 3-4

Ingredients

4 lbs. of beef short ribs

1 cup of unsweetened cranberry juice

2 tablespoons of apple-cider vinegar

Sea salt to taste

1 tablespoon of coconut oil

1½ cups of bone broth

1 cup of fresh cranberries

1 bay leaf

2 tablespoons of fresh parsley

Directions:

1. Meanwhile, you heat your oven to 300 degrees.
2. After which you heat the coconut oil in a heavy-bottomed pot (ideally cast iron) and brown the meat on all sides.
3. After that, you turn off the heat, remove the meat, and salt it.
4. Then you add the bone broth, cranberry juice, cranberries, cider vinegar, bay leaf and meat to the pot.
5. Remember, the liquid should come up to about ⅓ of the height of the meat - if any less, I suggest you add a little bit more broth or water.
6. Furthermore, making sure you have lid that fits tightly, braise for about 2-3 hours in the oven, checking periodically that there is enough liquid (**NOTE:** you shouldn't have a problem if the lid seals well).
7. Finally, you remove and cover the meat, strain the liquid and reduce about ½.
8. Then you garnish with fresh parsley

Beef and Butternut Stew with Pear and Thyme
Serves: 4-6

Ingredients

2-3 pound of roast or stew meat (for me I used sirloin tip) cut into 1½" cubes

5 cloves garlic (minced)

2 cups of bone broth

¼ teaspoon of cinnamon

2 pears (chopped)

1 tablespoon of fresh thyme

1½ tablespoons of coconut oil

1 onion (chopped)

2 inch piece ginger (minced)

1 cup of mushrooms (sliced)

½ teaspoon of sea salt

1 butternut squash (peeled and cubed)

Directions:

1. First, you heat 1 tablespoon of the coconut oil in a heavy-bottomed pot on medium-high heat and brown the meat on all sides.
2. After which you remove from the pot, and turn the heat down to medium.
3. After that, you add the onion and cook for about five minutes or until they begin to soften.
4. Then you add the ginger and garlic, and cook for another couple of minutes, being careful to stir them gently so that they don't burn.
5. At this point, you add the bone broth or stock and the browned meat to the pot, and bring to a simmer on low.
6. This is when you cover tightly and cook for 15 minutes, making sure to keep it at a simmer.
7. Furthermore, you add the butternut squash, cinnamon, and sea salt and simmer covered another 15 minutes.
8. This is the point, you add the pears and simmer for another 30 minutes, or until the meat and squash are both tender.

9. In a small skillet, you heat the rest of the coconut oil on high heat and cook the mushrooms for about 5 minutes, or until browned and tender.
10. Finally, when the stew is done, garnish with sautéed mushrooms and fresh thyme.

Three-Herb Beef Breakfast Patties
Serves: 6-8

Ingredients

1 tablespoon of fresh rosemary

1 tablespoon of fresh sage

1 tablespoon of coconut oil

2lbs of grass-fed ground beef

1 teaspoon of sea salt

1 tablespoon of fresh thyme

Directions:

1. First, in a large bowl, combine the ground beef, fresh herbs, and sea salt.
2. After which you form into patties using the palms of your hands.
3. After that, you heat some of the coconut oil in a cast-iron skillet on medium heat.
4. Then you cook the patties for about 5-8 minutes a side, until nicely browned on the outside and cooked throughout.

Perfect Pressure-Cooked Beef

Serves: 6-8

Ingredients

1 3-4 pound of beef roast (I used chuck)

A few sprigs of fresh herbs (I prefer to use a combo of rosemary and thyme)

1 tablespoon of coconut oil

1 cup of bone broth or better still water

1 tablespoon of apple-cider vinegar

Salt

Directions:

1. First, you heat the coconut oil in the pressure cooker and brown the meat.
2. After which you add the bone broth, cider vinegar, vinegar, herbs, and salt.
3. After that, you make sure the liquid comes up to ⅓ of the level of the meat; if not, add some water until it does.
4. Then you close the lid and bring the cooker to full pressure.
5. At this point, you cook for 35 minutes at pressure.
6. When it is finished, I suggest you let the pressure release naturally (**NOTE:** if you release pressure too quickly it may toughen the meat).
7. Remember that the meat should be able to be shredded easily with a fork.
8. Feel free to serve as-is or shred and add seasonings to put on salads, lettuce tacos, etc.

Pineapple-Marinated Steak

Serves: 4

Ingredients

2 tablespoons of fish sauce

1 teaspoon of sea salt

1½ lbs. of beef steak

1 cup of fresh pineapple chunks

2 tablespoons of coconut aminos

1 teaspoon of powdered ginger

½ teaspoon of garlic powder

Directions:

1. First, you combine pineapple, coconut aminos, fish sauce, salt, ginger, and garlic powder in a blender.
2. After which you pulse until smooth.
3. After that, you place steak in a large sealed plastic bag, add marinade, turn to coat.
4. Then you let marinate for at least 30 minutes (longer for tougher cuts of steak).
5. At this point, you heat grill to medium-high.
6. Furthermore, you remove steak from marinade (discard marinade) and quickly rinse steak.
7. Finally, you pat dry and grill, 4 to 6 minutes per side for medium-rare.
8. This is when you let rest for at least 5 minutes before slicing.
9. Make sure you add salt to taste.

Note: however, pineapple enzymes are powerful in breaking down protein, so be sure not to allow the steak to sit too long in marinade and follow the quick rinsing step

Pineapple Salsa-Stuffed Burgers

Serves: 2 burgers

Ingredients

Pineapple Salsa:

⅓ Cup of red onions (diced)

2 teaspoons of extra virgin olive oil

¼ teaspoon of sea salt

1½ cups of pineapples (diced)

¼ cup of cilantro (chopped)

1 tablespoon of lime juice

Burgers:

1 tablespoon of coconut oil

½ cup of pineapple salsa

1 pound of ground beef

¼ teaspoon of sea salt

Directions:

Directions for the salsa:

1. First, you combine all ingredients in a bowl and marinate in the fridge for at least 30 minutes.
2. Meanwhile, you heat the oven to 400 degrees F.
3. After that, you combine the meat and salt by hand and form into four balls, then flatten into ¼-inch thick patties.
4. After which you place half of the salsa on one of the patties and lay another patty on top.
5. Then you seal the edges by hand, making one large, fat burger.
6. Finally, you repeat for the remaining patties and salsa.

Meatballs in Sticky Peach Sauce
Serves: 4 to 6 servings

Ingredients

1 pound of ground pork

1 tablespoon of minced fresh rosemary

¾ teaspoon of fine sea salt

1 pound of ground beef

3 tablespoons of no-sugar-added peach preserves (homemade or better still store-bought)

1 teaspoon of dried thyme leaves

Directions:

1. First, you combine all meatball ingredients together in a large mixing bowl with your hands until evenly distributed.
2. After which you form 2-tablepoon-sized meatballs and place directly in a large skillet set over the stovetop.

NOTE: you will be able to fit the most meatballs if you place them in a concentric pattern.

3. Then once all the meatballs have been placed in the skillet, I suggest you turn the heat to medium-high.
4. At this point, you cook for 6 minutes until browned on the bottom, turn over with a spoon and cook an additional 5 to 6 minutes until slightly pink in the center.
5. This is when you turn off the heat and stir the meatballs to coat them in the pan juices.
6. Furthermore, you spoon the Sticky Peach Sauce on top of the meatballs.
7. After that, you broil for 4 to 5 minutes until the sauce has caramelized.
8. Finally, you serve warm over mashed parsnips or white sweet potatoes with the sauce spooned on top!

Zuppa Toscana
Serves: 4-6 servings

Ingredients

1 small onion (chopped)

2 cloves garlic (minced)

1 large celeriac (peeled and chopped)

⅓ Cup of coconut milk

6 slices bacon

1 lb. of ground beef

4 cups of bone broth

2 cups of kale (chopped)

Directions:

1. First, you cook the bacon in a stock pot over medium heat until crispy, and then remove it from the pan, leaving the bacon fat behind.
2. After which you add the onion and cook for about 3 minutes until translucent.
3. After that, you add the ground beef and cook, stirring, for about 3 minutes until browned.
4. At this point, you add the garlic and cook, stirring, another 2-3 minutes.
5. This is when you add the broth and celeriac and bring to a boil.
6. Furthermore, you reduce the heat to a simmer and cook, uncovered, 20 minutes or until the celeriac is tender.
7. After that, you add the kale and coconut milk and cook until the kale wilts.
8. Finally, you serve topped with crumbled bacon.

Pan-Fried Pork Medallions with Sage and Cream
Serves: 4

Ingredients

1 tablespoon of lard or better still other solid fat

¾ cup of coconut cream

4 teaspoon of coconut aminos

1 tablespoon of chopped sage leaves

2 (about 1¾ lb.) pork fillets, trimmed

½ cup of chicken bone broth

½ teaspoon of fish sauce

1 teaspoon of lemon juice

Directions:

1. First, you trim the pork fillets of any membrane and slice into 1½ inch rounds, to yield around 3 per person.
2. After which you heat a frying pan on medium heat and melt the lard.
3. Then when the pan is hot, add the pork pieces (cut side down) and cook for around 3-4 minutes on either side, or until just cooked through.
4. After that, you regulate the stove temperature if you feel it is getting too hot.
5. At this point, you remove pork to a warmed plate, along with the juices.
6. This is when you pour the broth into the pan and scrape the bottom to release any sediment into the sauce.
7. Furthermore, you add the cream and bring everything up to a simmer.
8. After that, you add the fish sauce, coconut aminos, lemon juice, sage and the meat juices.
9. Then you taste and sprinkle in a little salt if necessary, but it probably won't be.
10. Finally, you divide the pork between warmed plates and spoon the sauce over top.

Notes

I prefer to serve this with zucchini ribbons sautéed in a little fat, but it is equally delicious over caulimash/rice.

Moroccan-Inspired Breakfast Skillet

Serves: 4 servings

Ingredients

2 tablespoons of solid cooking fat (coconut oil or better still lard work well here)

One small bunch chard stems removed, separated, and both stems and leaves chopped

1 teaspoon of ground turmeric

⅛ Teaspoon of cinnamon

½ cup of raisins

1 lb. of pastured ground pork

1 (about 2 cups) medium sweet potato, diced

3 cloves garlic (minced)

½ teaspoon of sea salt

1 teaspoon apple cider vinegar

Directions:

1. First, you place the ground pork in the bottom of a cold heavy-bottomed pan, and break up slightly with a utensil.
2. After which you turn on medium-high heat, and cook, stirring, until the meat is browned and has absorbed all of the fat (NOTE: don't drain it off!).
3. After that, you turn off the heat, transfer to a large bowl and set aside.
4. Then you place the same pan back on the stove, add the solid cooking fat, and turn the heat to medium-high.
5. At this point, when the fat has melted and the pan is hot, add the sweet potatoes and cook, stirring, for five minutes.
6. This is when you add the chard stems and cook for three more minutes.
7. Furthermore, you add the garlic, turmeric, sea salt, and cinnamon, and stir to combine.
8. After which you cook for a few more minutes, until the sweet potatoes are just soft.
9. Then you add the chard leaves, apple cider vinegar, and raisins to the pan.
10. In addition, you continue cooking until chard has wilted, about a minute or two.
11. Finally, you turn off the heat, salt to taste, and serve warm!

Pork Roast with Balsamic Reduction

Serves: 16 servings

Ingredients

1 cup of balsamic vinegar

½ tablespoon of sea salt

½ teaspoon of dried sage

4-lb of pork roast

¼ cup of maple syrup

½ tablespoon of dried rosemary

½ teaspoon of dried thyme

Directions:

1. First, you combine all ingredients in a slow cooker and cook on low for 8-10 hours, until the meat is easily shredded with a fork.
2. After which you strain the liquid into a saucepan and bring to a boil, then reduce the heat to a simmer.
3. After that, you reduce the liquid by half, about 15 minutes.
4. Then you serve the sliced or shredded pork topped with the sauce.

Meatballs in Sticky Peach Sauce
Serves: 4 to 6 servings

Ingredients

1 pound of ground pork

1 tablespoon of minced fresh rosemary

¾ teaspoon of fine sea salt

1 pound of ground beef

3 tablespoons of no-sugar-added peach preserves (homemade or store-bought)

1 teaspoon of dried thyme leaves

Directions:

1. First, you combine all meatball ingredients together in a large mixing bowl with your hands until evenly distributed.
2. After which you form 2-tablepoon-sized meatballs and place directly in a large skillet set over the stovetop.

NOTE: you will be able to fit the most meatballs if you place them in a concentric pattern.

3. Then once all the meatballs have been placed in the skillet, turn the heat to medium-high.
4. After that, you cook for 6 minutes until browned on the bottom, turn over with a spoon and cook an additional 5 to 6 minutes until slightly pink in the center.
5. This is when you turn off the heat and stir the meatballs to coat them in the pan juices.
6. Furthermore, you spoon the Sticky Peach Sauce on top of the meatballs.
7. At this point, you broil for 4 to 5 minutes until the sauce has caramelized.
8. Finally, you serve warm over mashed parsnips or white sweet potatoes with the sauce spooned on top!

Thai-Inspired Pork Salad
Serves: 2 servings

Ingredients

1 lb. of ground pork

2 large cloves garlic (peeled and thinly sliced)

Zest and juice of one large lime

1 tablespoon of fish sauce

½ packed cup of cilantro leaves (chopped)

1 tablespoon of lard or better still other solid fat

1 1/2-inch piece ginger (peeled and finely grated)

5 shallots (peeled and thinly sliced)

4 green onions (thinly sliced on the diagonal)

1 tablespoon of coconut aminos

½ packed cup Thai basil leaves (chopped)

¼ packed cup mint leaves (chopped)

Extra lime wedges to serve

Directions:

1. First, you heat the fat on a fairly high heat in a large skillet or wok and tip in the pork.
2. After which you cook for 4-5 minutes until the liquid has all but evaporated and the pork is beginning to brown.
3. Whilst this is happening, I suggest you break down the ground meat's tendency to clump with a long handled wooden fork or spoon.
4. After that, you add the ginger, garlic and shallots and cook for 3 minutes, stirring very frequently.

NOTE: you want the pork to crisp up but not burn on the bottom of the pan so I suggest you keep that fork/spoon moving.

5. At this point, you stir in the lime zest and juice, together with the green onions, and cook a further minute.

6. This is when you tip in the fish sauce and coconut aminos and cook one minute more, scraping the sediment off the bottom of the pan all the while.
7. Finally, you remove from the heat, throw in the herbs, give it all a good mix and serve with a decent wedge of lime on the side.

Notes

Delicious hot, warm or cold, I suggest you served with kelp noodles or in lettuce boats. With noodles included, this recipe serves 3.

Pork Pesto Skillet

Serves: 4 servings

Ingredients

½ cup of extra virgin olive oil

1 clove garlic

1 bunch kale

2 lbs. of ground pork

2 cups of fresh basil, tightly packed (about the contents of a 4-oz container)

1 lemon (juiced)

½ teaspoon of sea salt

Directions:

1. First, you gently pre-heat a skillet on medium-high heat for a minute.
2. Then when it is ready, add the ground pork, breaking up in to bits and cooking for 10-15 minutes, stirring, until browned.
3. Meanwhile, you place the olive oil, basil, garlic, lemon juice, and salt into a blender.
4. After which you blend for 30 seconds or just until incorporated (or more, if you like a more blended pesto).

NOTE: you may need to use your tamper here, or stop the blender to scrape the sides down-- whatever works!

5. Then once the pork has reabsorbed all of the fat and started browning, I suggest you add the kale to the skillet and continue cooking for a few minutes, being sure to stir occasionally.
6. Finally, you turn off the heat and add the pesto to the skillet. Stir to combine and serve warm.

Veggie-Lover's Meatza
Serves: 8-12 servings

Ingredients

1 teaspoon of sea salt

1 teaspoon of ground ginger

½ cup of your favorite AIP-friendly "tomato" sauce or better still BBQ sauce

½ yellow squash (sliced)

3 ounces olives (sliced)

3 pounds of ground meat

1 teaspoon of dried oregano

1 dash ground cinnamon

½ zucchini (sliced)

4 ounces mushrooms (sliced)

Directions:

1. Meanwhile, you heat the oven to 350 degrees F.
2. After which you combine the ground meat and spices and mix well.
3. After that, you line a rimmed baking sheet with parchment paper or a silicone liner.
4. At this point, you spread the meat over the sheet, flattening it evenly to about ¼ inch.
5. Then you bake for 10 minutes or until cooked through.
6. This is when you transfer to a pizza stone or a wire rack on top of a baking sheet.
7. Finally, you add the sauce and toppings, then return to the oven for 10 minutes or until the toppings are cooked.

Italian-Spiced 50/50 Sausages

Serves: 8-10 patties

Ingredients

1 pound of pastured ground pork

1 tablespoon of minced fresh thyme

½ teaspoon of garlic powder

1 tablespoon of solid cooking fat (lards, coconut oil tallow, or duck fat)

1 pound of grass-fed ground beef

1 tablespoon of minced fresh oregano

1 tablespoon of minced fresh parsley (it is optional)

½ teaspoon of sea salt

Directions:

1. First, you place the pork, herbs, ground beef, garlic powder and salt in a large bowl and combine well with your hands.
2. After which you form into 8-10 patties and place on a plate.
3. After that, you heat the solid cooking fat in the bottom of a cast-iron skillet or frying pan on medium heat.
4. Then when the fat is melted and the pan is hot, add patties, cook 10 minutes a side, or until thoroughly cooked.

NOTE: you may have to do this in two batches. Alternately, you can bake them at 400 degrees for 20 minutes or until they are cooked throughout.

Variation: you can switch up the protein in these--you can make them 100% beef or pork, or add some lamb into the mix!

Serves: 6-8 as a side dish

Ingredients

1 cup of fresh cranberries (cut into halves)

4 slices of pastured bacon

4 stalks celery (chopped)

2 tablespoons of rosemary (minced)

2 cups of mushrooms (sliced thinly)

1 green apple (cut into 1" squares)

½ teaspoon of sea salt

1 sweet potato (cut into 1" squares)

¾ cup of bone broth

½ onions (chopped)

4 cloves garlic (minced)

1 tablespoon of solid cooking fat

¼ teaspoon of cinnamon

1½ heads of cauliflower (processed in a food processor until it forms "rice" sized granules)

Directions:

1. Meanwhile, you heat your oven to 350 degrees.
2. After which you combine the sweet potatoes, cranberries, and bone broth in a large baking dish.
3. After that, you bake in the oven for 30 minutes, stirring once to ensure even cooking.
4. In the meantime, you cook the bacon slices in a skillet on medium heat, turning when needed, until they are crispy.
5. When they are finished, I suggest you remove and let cool, leaving the fat in the pan.
6. Furthermore, you add the onion and celery, and cook for 8 minutes, or until beginning to brown.
7. At this point, you add the garlic and rosemary, and cook for another couple of minutes.

8. This is when you remove the onion mixture from the pan into a small bowl and set aside.
9. In addition, you add the solid cooking fat and the mushrooms to the pan.
10. After which you cook, stirring, for a couple of minutes until the mushrooms are browned.
11. After that, you add the cauliflower "rice", and cook, stirring for five minutes; set aside.
12. Then when the sweet potato mixture is finished cooking, you remove from the oven and turn the heat up to 425 degrees.
13. This is when you add the cauliflower mixture; the onion mixture, the apple as well as the cinnamon and sea salt to the sweet potato mixture and stir to combine.
14. Finally, you place back in the oven for another 10 minutes. Let cool for a few minutes, and serve warm.

Note: If you are using this to stuff a turkey, I suggest you skip the last 10 minutes of cooking - it will have plenty of time in the oven with the bird!

Celeriac Leek Soup
Serves: 4

Ingredients

2 leeks (ends removed and sliced thinly)

1-inch piece ginger (minced)

2 pounds of celeriac (peeled and cut into 1 ½ inch chunks)

4 slices of sugar-free (pastured bacon)

3 cloves garlic (minced)

4 cups of bone broth

1 tablespoon of apple-cider vinegar

½ teaspoon of salt

A few sprigs of parsley

Directions:

1. First, you heat a heavy-bottomed pot on medium heat; when it is ready, cook the bacon until crispy, turning a couple times.
2. After which you remove the bacon to cool and leave the fat in the bottom of the pan.
3. After that, you add the leeks and cook for a few minutes, stirring.
4. Then you add the garlic and ginger and cook for another couple of minutes.
5. At this point, you add the broth, celeriac, apple-cider vinegar and salt and bring to a boil.
6. This is when you turn down to a simmer, cover, and cook for 15 minutes, or until celeriac is soft.
7. Furthermore, while the soup is cooking, crumble the bacon.
8. At this point, you transfer to a blender and process until desired consistency is reached, adding more bone broth if needed.
9. Finally, you serve with parsley and crumbled bacon on top.

CONCLUSION

The Autoimmune Fix Diet Cookbook, will show you a breakthrough plan to stop auto-immune triggers and restore your health.

If you followed this book judiciously, it has what it takes to bring your athletic performance back to an admirable height. I suggest you give it a trial.

Remember, the only bad action you can take is no action at all.

Made in the USA
San Bernardino, CA
26 November 2016